ANESTHESIA AND THE PATIENT WITH HEART DISEASE

ANESTHESIA AND THE PATIENT WITH HEART DISEASE

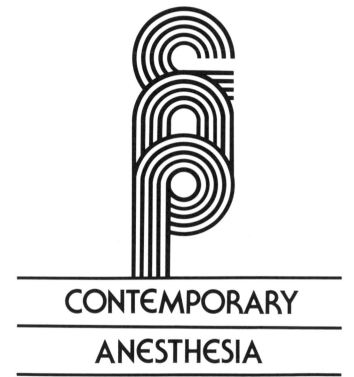

CONTEMPORARY

ANESTHESIA

PRACTICE

BURNELL R. BROWN, JR., EDITOR

CASEY D. BLITT & A.H. GIESECKE, ASSOCIATE EDITORS

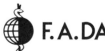 F.A. DAVIS COMPANY/PHILADELPHIA

Library of Congress Cataloging in Publication Data
Main entry under title:

Anesthesia and the patient with heart disease.

    (Contemporary anesthesia practice; v. 2)
    Bibliography: p.
    Includes index.
    1. Anesthesia—Complications and sequelae. 2. Heart
—Diseases—Complications and sequelae. I. Brown, Burnell R. II.
Series. [DNLM: 1. Anesthetics—Pharmacodynamics. 2. Anesthesia. 3.
Heart—Drug effects. W1 C0769ME v. 2 / W0460 A579]
RD87.3.H43A5   617'.96   79-17989
ISBN 0-8036-1260-5

PREFACE

Preservation of circulation and ventilation are the two prime concerns of the anesthesiologist. Advances in knowledge of circulatory physiology have been made in Brobdingnagian fashion in the past decade, with new concepts introduced that are quite adaptable to the clinical sphere. Knowledge has reversed anesthetic dictums 180 degrees in certain cases. Cyclopropane used to enjoy the reputation of the king of anesthetics in patients with peripheral circulatory collapse caused by hypervolemia and in those with failing myocardiums; thus, use was based on one circulatory variable, the blood pressure, which seemed better preserved with cyclopropane than with other anesthetics. Cyclopropane has now fallen into disrepute, not only because of flammability, but because it is now recognized that maintenance of blood pressure with the drug is due to its profound stimulation of the sympathetic nervous system. Exaggerated sympathetic tone is now considered an anathema in shock states because of the resultant hypoperfusion of certain vital organs. Other concepts are changing. Morphine anesthesia was shown to have minimal cardiac and peripheral vascular actions, yet this very lack of negative inotropic effect may cause greater myocardial consumption of oxygen in the patient anesthetized with

v

morphine than in the patient deeply anesthetized with halothane. The adage that the questions remain the same over the years but the answers change is quite true.

Volume 2 of Contemporary Anesthesia Practice is designed for rapid reading and assimilation by the practicing anesthetist of new developments and various procedures in managing the anesthesia of a patient with cardiac disease for noncardiac surgery. It is not intended to be authoritative, but simply suggests lines of management and treatment of patients as seen on a day-to-day basis. This volume consists of a potpourri of articles, each developing a theme that, it is hoped, will be of practical value. Theoretic considerations and irrelevant research have been held to a minimum. It is the ultimate aspiration of the Editor that this text will contribute to better care of patients.

Burnell R. Brown, Jr., M.D., Ph.D.

CONTRIBUTORS

Hugh D. Allen, M.D.
Associate Professor
Department of Pediatrics
Section of Pediatric Cardiology
University of Arizona College of Medicine
Tucson, Arizona

John L. Atlee, III, M.D.
Associate Professor
Department of Anesthesiology
University of Wisconsin Medical Center
Madison, Wisconsin

Casey D. Blitt, M.D.
Associate Professor
Department of Anesthesiology
University of Arizona College of Medicine
Tucson, Arizona

Burnell R. Brown, Jr., M.D., Ph.D.
Professor and Head
Department of Anesthesiology
University of Arizona College of Medicine
Tucson, Arizona

Gordon A. Ewy, M.D.
Professor
Department of Internal Medicine
Director, Diagnostic Cardiology
University of Arizona College of Medicine

Joseph C. Gabel, M.D.
Professor
Department of Anesthesiology
University of Texas Medical Branch
Galveston, Texas

G. Y. Gaines, M.D.
Assistant Professor
Department of Anesthesiology
University of Texas Southwestern Medical School at Dallas
Dallas, Texas

A. H. Giesecke, Jr., M.D.
Jenkins Professor
Department of Anesthesiology
University of Texas Southwestern Medical School at Dallas
Dallas, Texas

Richard B. Knapp, M.D.
Chairman and Professor
Department of Anesthesiology
West Virginia University Medical Center
Morgantown, West Virginia

Robert G. Merin, M.D.
Professor
Department of Anesthesiology
University of Rochester Medical Center
Rochester, New York

John H. Tinker, M.D.
Assistant Professor of Anesthesiology
Mayo Medical School and Mayo Clinic
Rochester, Minnesota

Alan S. Tonnesen, M.D.
Associate Professor
Department of Anesthesiology
University of Texas Medical Branch
Galveston, Texas

CONTENTS

EFFECTS OF ANESTHETICS AND ANESTHETIC ADJUVANTS ON THE HEART

Robert G. Merin, M.D.

Dr. Merin discusses the effects of inhalation anesthetics and injectable drugs on myocardial performance. A real clinical dilemma is created by the intrinsic negative inotropic action of the anesthetics. Reduction in diastolic pressure decreases coronary perfusion, but there is also a decrease in the need and utilization of oxygen by myocardial fiber, simultaneously. Do these effects parallel one another or are they disparate? Accumulating evidence indicates that consumption of oxygen may decline to a somewhat greater extent than myocardial blood flow. Obviously, this is optimal if correct. Such observations could lead to greater utilization of anesthetics such as halothane and enflurane during surgery in the patient with coronary artery disease.

Burnell R. Brown, Jr.

The basic function of the heart is to provide the driving force for perfusion and nourishment of the various organ systems of the body and to carry away the products of metabolism and of organ function (e.g., carbon dioxide, water, nitrogen). The heart, then, functions as a pump, whose output depends on the rate at which it beats and the ventricular function during each cardiac cycle. In considering the effect of anesthetics on cardiac function, I shall work in the framework of these two aspects. I shall discuss the perfusion and metabolism of the heart to a certain extent and will briefly review what we know about the effect of anesthetics on these aspects of cardiac function, predominantly in man.

Heart Rate and Rhythm

Although the rate of cardiac contraction is depressed in a dose-related manner by anesthetics in isolated hearts or heart-lung preparations,[1] the effect in intact animals and in man is less predictable. This results from the fact that the heart rate in the intact animal is determined largely by the relationship between the sympathetic and parasympathetic nervous effect on the heart. Man's slow heart rate at rest (60 to 80 beats per minute) is a result of tonic vagal (parasympathetic) stimulation slowing the faster intrinsic rate (100 to 120 beats per minute) of the normal cardiac pacemaker, the sinoatrial node. Conversely, tachycardias are a result of the stimulation of the sympathetic nervous system overriding the vagal effects. Naturally, then, the effect on heart rate of anesthetics is largely related to influence on the autonomic nervous system in the intact animal.[2] Therefore, the state of the patient or volunteer in the studies of the effect of anesthetics on man is also important. If there is a high resting heart rate, then the anesthetic will tend to decrease it. If the heart rate is low in the resting state with vagal predominance, then often the anesthetic will tend to increase the heart rate. The reflex control of cardiac function is mediated through the various baroreceptors throughout the body, located in both high pressure (aortic and carotid) and low pressure (atrial and vena caval) systems.[3] They provide the afferent limb, which is integrated in the central nervous system to modulate the autonomic nervous influences of the heart. The effect of anesthetics on this aspect of the control of heart rate (and ventricular function) is not clear at the present time. In addition, circulating catecholamines from the adrenal medulla also affect heart rate (and occasionally rhythm), and anesthetics may influence adrenal medullary catecholamine release.

Ventricular Function

Although this review will concentrate on the effect of anesthetics on ventricular function in man, it is necessary to consider briefly some aspects of in vitro cardiac muscle mechanics.[4, 5] All muscle can function in two basic fashions, isometrically and isotonically. In a muscle bath, resting muscle length is determined by the weight or load placed on the muscle strip (preload). This can be precisely regulated in the experimental condition. In the isometric contraction, the muscle fiber length is fixed, so that during a muscle contraction there is no change in length, but rather tension is developed. During an isotonic contraction, the muscle is loaded (afterload) and allowed to shorten during stimulation, thus performing external work by moving the applied load. The rate and degree of tension developed (isometric), the speed of shortening, the distance moved, and the load carried (isotonic) can be directly measured in the isolated muscle preparation. Through this sort of investigation, it is well established that there are a number of influences on the function of the heart muscle. The first influence is the resting length of the muscle, which is determined by the load applied to the muscle, the preload. As preload increases up to a certain point, the contractile function of the muscle also increases. The second important influence is afterload. In an isotonic contraction, the higher the load that the muscle must move (with all other factors remaining constant), the less will be the contractile performance of the isolated muscle. The third factor that influences muscular performance is the rate of stimulation. Again, within certain limits, the higher the rate of stimulation, the greater will be the contractile performance of the muscle. Finally, the environment in which the isolated muscle contracts is an important determinant of performance. Hypoxia, increase in hydrogen ion concentration, absence of nutrients, presence of neurohumors and hormones, and, of course, added drugs will have a major effect on the performance of the muscle in vitro.

In the intact animal (including man), one can also consider

various phases of the cardiac cycle as being analogous to those of isolated muscle. However, quantitation of the performance of the intact heart is more difficult and less precise than in isolated muscle and subject to more extraneous influences. Isovolumic contraction occurs between the time that activation of the ventricle begins and the outflow valves (pulmonary and aortic) open. This period is analogous to isometric contraction in isolated muscle and can be measured in man and the intact animal by the development of tension between two pedestals of a strain gauge arch sutured to the epicardial surface of the ventricle or by events occurring in the ventricle before the outflow valves open, such as pressure development indices (dP/dt) or the time intervals (the pre-ejection period—PEP).[6] After the outflow valves open, the pumping function of the heart can be viewed as isotonic contractile performance. Estimates of this aspect of ventricular function include the measurement of blood flow (and acceleration) by flow meters; measurement of the output of the ventricle (stroke volume) by various means, including dye dilution, thermal dilution, and direct Fick techniques; the ejection time indices, such as left ventricular ejection time (LVET); and other indirect reflections of the pumping function of the heart, such as the IJ wave of the ballistocardiogram (BCG).

All these measures are more or less dependent on the same factors that influence the contractile function in isolated muscle. The ease and accuracy of measurement of these factors, just as with ventricular performance, is not as simple in intact animals. The following methods for estimating these influences in man are listed in order of decreasing precision.

Preload

The best estimate of preload in the intact heart is the end-diastolic fiber length, which is best measured by end-diastolic volume. This is a difficult measurement at the present time, and usually, even in the catheterization laboratory, ventricular end-diastolic pressure is used to approximate preload. In the clinical situation, even this is rarely measured. During cardiovascular surgery, atrial pressures are frequently measured. If the integrity of the chest is intact, then the best measure of the left ventricular preload is undoubtedly the pulmonary artery occluded pressure (PAOP) or wedge pressure, which reflects left atrial pressure fairly accurately.[7] For estimates of right heart function, the central venous pressure bears the same relationship to right ventricular filling pressures as pulmonary artery occluded pressure does to left ventricular filling pressures. However, it must be noted that if the left ventricle is being studied, measures of the right ventricular filling pressure may not be the appropriate measurement.

Afterload

There is some evidence to suggest that the effects of afterload on isometric and isotonic contraction are somewhat different. Increasing afterload when one is measuring isovolumic performance of the ventricle tends to increase the maximum rate of pressure development within limits. Consequently, increasing afterload can increase these estimates of ventricular function without other changes in ventricular performance. As for the pumping function of the heart, there is reasonably good evidence to suggest that as in isotonic contraction and isolated muscle, the greater the afterload, the lower the pumping function of the heart. Likewise, measurement of afterload in the intact animal should be somewhat different for the two types of contraction.[8] For isovolumic (isometric) contractile function, aortic blood pressure is a reasonable estimate of afterload. However, for estimates of effects of afterload on the pumping function of the heart (isotonic), vascular resistance in the systemic bed and vascular impedance in the pulmonary bed are the best estimates. If these are not available, then arterial pressure is a rough gauge for both.

Rate of Stimulation

Measurement of heart rate is relatively easy and accurate.

Environment of the Muscle

Ideally, one should measure the concentrations of all factors in the blood perfusing the heart that might influence contractile function. This certainly includes pH, pO_2, and pCO_2. In addition, the concentration of the drug being studied should be measured in some fashion. Finally, in order to be sure about direct effects of interventions, the effect of the autonomic nervous system (particularly the sympathetic nervous system) ideally should be documented. Increasing precision of measurement of blood catecholamines may facilitate our understanding of this influence, although in the past mixed venous or arterial catecholamine concentrations have been of limited value.

Certainly, the most common method of measuring ventricular function in man has been to measure cardiac output. There can be little question about the dependence of cardiac output on the factors that have been just outlined. In fact, one of the more precise methods of measuring cardiac output is to graph preload against some measure of ventricular performance.[9] Such ventricular function curves are easy to produce in heart-lung preparations, more difficult to develop in the intact animal, and very difficult to measure in man. However, the principle should be adhered to when considering the meaning of measurements of cardiac output. The influences of heart rate, preload, and afterload are well known, and these should at least be measured, in order to estimate their influence on the other measurements being performed. Although many more precise measures of ventricular function have been touted over the years, in fact, there is no measure that is free of the influence of the factors previously noted. This means that in order to precisely know what the effect of an intervention or drug is on ventricular function in man, these factors should be measured during the course of the experiment.

EFFECTS OF ANESTHETICS

Heart Rate and Rhythm

Inasmuch as heart rate in man is controlled by the interaction between the sympathetic and parasympathetic nervous system, the effect of anesthetics on the autonomic nervous system is largely responsible for changes in heart rate. Until recently, it appeared that anesthetics could be separated into two distinct groups, according to their effect on the autonomic nervous system.[10] So-called Group 1 anesthetics, which include diethyl ether, cyclopropane and fluroxene, appeared to produce stimulation of the sympathetic nervous system, which tended to antagonize the direct depressant effects of these drugs on ventricular function (see following section). Presumably, this effect would also result in increasing heart rate. Group 2 anesthetics, such as halothane, methoxyflurane, enflurane, and barbiturates, produced little sympathetic stimulation, and the end-result was a dose-related depressant effect on ventricular function in the intact animal. However, the categorization appears to be more complicated. In terms of effects on heart rate, although heart rate is increased with both diethyl ether[11, 12] and fluroxene[13] as might be expected, there is no consistent change with cyclopropane in man.[14, 15] In addition, although heart rate does not change with halothane as one might predict,[16, 17, 18] with methoxyflurane,[19] enflurane,[20, 21] and isoflurane[22] there is a significant and often marked increase in heart rate during anesthesia. With isoflurane, this positive chronotropic action appears to be dose-related. During clinical anesthesia and surgery, the direct effects of anesthetics on heart rate appear to be less important than the environmental changes produced by instrumentation and surgical procedures.[23] All anesthetics can produce direct effects on conduction of cardiac impulse, especially through the atrioventricular nodal system. However, these effects on the function of the heart have not been well outlined.

Ventricular Function

Although all potent anesthetics depress cardiac function in vitro (muscle strips or perfused heart), several appear to have minimal depressive actions in the intact animal and man. As mentioned, these anesthetics presumably produce stimulation of the sympathetic nervous system. However, they are of historical significance primarily, for diethyl ether, cyclopropane, and fluroxene are rarely used clinically today. Studies in man have indicated with all three anesthetics that, even at relatively high concentrations, cardiac output was not decreased when compared with the awake state.[11-15] With diethyl ether and cyclopropane, this was partly a consequence of an increasing heart rate. However, in several instances there were minimal changes in stroke volume as well. In addition, the IJ wave of the BCG was not depressed with fluroxene and even increased at the highest concentration, possibly as a result of the marked increase in heart rate.[13] In none of the studies was there an adequate estimate of preload, with either right atrial or central venous pressure being the only measurement. Of particular interest is the demonstration of the importance of sympathetic nervous activity in the maintenance of ventricular function with diethyl ether and cyclopropane. Beta-adrenergic receptor blockade with propranolol resulted in marked decrease in stroke volume and increase in central venous pressure during diethyl ether anesthesia.[24] Local anesthetic blockade of the cervical sympathetic ganglia during cyclopropane anesthesia in man resulted in much the same effect.[25]

HALOTHANE

Halothane is by far the most widely studied of the inhalation anesthetics in animal and man. Dose-related depression of isometric function in man by halothane has been documented by use of a strain gauge arch sewn to the ventricular epicardium during surgery,[26] and by depression of left ventricular indices during anesthesia alone.[27] Decreased isotonic ventricular performance has been documented repeatedly by using various techniques of measuring cardiac output.[16-18, 27] In addition, systolic time intervals and the IJ wave of the BCG have also been studied.[17] Recently, changes in left ventricular filling pressures, measured by use of a pulmonary artery catheter[18] and direct left ventricular catheterization,[27] have been documented during halothane anesthesia. Increase in both pressures, together with the decreasing ventricular function as the halothane dose was increased, leaves little doubt that halothane produces a marked dose-related depression of ventricular function.

ENFLURANE

Early studies on the cardiovascular effects of enflurane in man were interpreted to mean that the drug produced minimal cardiovascular depression.[20, 21, 28] However, animal studies[29] and a carefully done experiment with human volunteers[30] indicate without question that the drug produces cardiac depression at least equivalent to that seen with halothane. Although the rise in preload accompanies depression of cardiac output, and the IJ wave of the BCG has not been documented, it appears likely that enflurane does produce a direct dose-related depression in ventricular function, similar to that seen with halothane.

ISOFLURANE

The delay in release of isoflurane for clinical use has slowed investigation of this interesting anesthetic. The original studies in man published in 1971 suggested that isoflurane produces minimal cardiovascular depression even at high concentrations.[22] However, this was at least in part a result of the rather marked increase in heart rate that was seen with these high concentrations. In addition, unlike halothane, a significant decrease in afterload (systemic vascular resistance) was also seen, which would lead to a positive effect on the pumping action of the heart. The effect of preload has not been adequately documented thus far. It would appear, however, that isoflurane does depress the heart in man less than its isomer enflurane and the cardiac depressant halothane.

NITROUS OXIDE

Since nitrous oxide is a relatively impotent central nervous system depressant, it has been generally considered to have minimal effects on other organ systems as well. However, recent studies have indicated that as little as 40 percent nitrous oxide can produce a small but significant depression in ventricular function in man.[31] In addition, nitrous oxide added to narcotic analgesics results in a more severe depression of ventricular function.[32] Finally, when added to potent inhalation anesthetics, a variety of effects have been seen (e.g., increased arterial pressure and systemic vascular resistance), suggesting a vasoconstrictive property of the drug.[33, 34] The mechanism and significance of these effects is still unclear at the moment, but suffice it to say that some thought must be given to the addition of nitrous oxide to more potent anesthetics in situations in which cardiac depression may be undesirable.

INTRAVENOUS ANESTHETICS

The sole use of an intravenous drug in order to produce effective surgical anesthesia is uncommon in clinical practice today. Rather, these drugs are used as adjuvants either to inhalation anesthetics or to one another, providing either analgesia, amnesia and hypnosis, or muscle relaxation. In spite of this fact, in most instances, the effect of the drugs has been studied separately rather than in combination, and I will review what is known about them.

HYPNOTICS AND AMNESICS

The time-tested and most popular of this group of drugs are the barbiturates. The ultra short-acting drugs (thiamylal, thiopental, methohexital) all appear to have much the same effect on the heart. Early work suggested that most of the depression of cardiac output seen with these drugs resulted from venodilation and decreased venous return to the heart, which produced inadequate diastolic filling.[35] More recent data using left ventricular dP/dt in man have shown small but significant depression in ventricular function, accompanied by some arterial hypotension and resultant tachycardia.[36]

Diazepam has been popular as both a premedicant and as an anesthetic adjuvant in recent years. Low doses (0.13 mg/kg) produce little effect on cardiac output, while large doses (0.77 mg/kg) result in a 30 percent decrease in stroke volume in healthy patients.[37]

Several intravenous induction agents not yet available in the United States have been tested in man. Propranidid (a eugenol derivative) has been in widespread use in Europe for 10 years. Recent data in man indicate that it produces significantly more depression on ventricular function than the barbiturates.[38] The synthetic steroid combination althesin appears to have effects on ventricular function similar to those of barbiturates, with perhaps slightly more tachycardia.[39] Etomidate is an imidazole-carboxyl ester, the latest of the new intravenous hypnotic drugs being investigated. Preliminary data in animal and man have indicated that it has the least cardiac depressant effect of any of the induction agents tested[40]; however, it must be used with other drugs because of a significant incidence of excess muscle activity in man. The future of this drug remains uncertain at the present time.

ANALGESICS

Although small doses of various narcotic analgesic drugs have been used as anesthetic supplements for a considerable period of time, there had been little investigation of the cardiovascular effects until Lowenstein and coworkers studied the effect of 1–2 mg/kg intravenous morphine on cardiac output and vascular pressures.[41] Their demonstration of no depression of ventricular function in a group of healthy patients and improvement in ventricular function in a group of patients with valvular heart disease began the era of the use of large doses of narcotic analgesics for anesthesia in man. Other studies have validated their results.[32] In addition, it has been demonstrated that nitrous oxide added to morphine anesthesia can result in significant depression of ventricular function.[32] Other narcotic analgesics have also been used, particularly the newer short-acting drugs, such as fentanyl.[42] Convincing evidence of a difference in effect on the cardiovascular system has not been forthcoming.

KETAMINE

One of the original attractions of ketamine was that it did not cause cardiovascular depression. In fact, ketamine appeared to increase ventricular function in healthy patients. The best of the published studies on the effect of anesthetics on ventricular function in man looked at the effect of 2 mg/kg ketamine in patients with angina pectoris without demonstrated coronary pathology by angiography.[43] This study showed a definite increase in both isometric (dP/dt/IP) and isotonic (cardiac output) function of the heart in man, with constant paced heart rate and no change in preload. In the clinical situation, however, there is a constant increase in heart rate with ketamine, which may also result in some decrease in stroke volume, although it still produces an increase in left ventricular dP/dt.

NEUROLEPTANESTHESIA

The combination of the butyrophenone derivative, droperidol, and the short-acting narcotic analgesic, fentanyl, was originally termed neuroleptanesthesia. However, much the same effects can be produced with other potent central nervous system drugs, such as the phenothiazines and the other narcotic analgesics. The original combination has been shown to have little effect on ventricular function in healthy man, although the studies published did not document preload effects. [42, 44, 45] Nevertheless, it appears that this combination generally preserves ventricular function in doses that produce conditions suitable for surgical anesthesia.

NEUROMUSCULAR BLOCKING DRUGS

Although it is difficult to measure the effect of these drugs by themselves (for obvious ethical reasons), all available studies have shown that none of the commonly employed agents (succinylcholine, d-tubocurarine, pancuronium, and gallamine) have an appreciable effect on ventricular function.[46-48] Two of these investigations employed the strain gauge arch sewn to the epicardium of patients during cardiopulmonary bypass.[46, 47] It must be remembered, however, that succinylcholine can produce bradycardia and/or ventricular arrhythmias, particularly in association with hyperkalemia and diseased states with marked tissue wasting (e.g., burns, paraplegia and other neurologic diseases, and massive trauma).[49] D-tubocurarine tends to produce bradycardia and hypotension, while gallamine and pancuronium generally cause an increase in heart rate and little change in arterial blood pressure.

REGIONAL ANESTHESIA

Local anesthetics have a direct effect on both cardiac rhythm and ventricular function in isolated hearts. However, the two effects can be dissociated, since the drugs are commonly used for arrhythmia treatment in animals and man. It is possible for enough local anesthetic to be absorbed into the systemic circulation to produce ventricular depression if large doses are used for the blocks (brachial plexus and epidural). However, with reasonable care concerning dose and method of injection, this risk should be minimal. If the nerve block includes a significant portion of the autonomic nervous system (spinal, epidural, and ninth and tenth cranial nerve), cardiac performance may be affected by the block itself. In healthy normovolemic man, epidural and spinal anesthesia to as high as the second thoracic dermatome produce minimal changes in the pumping function of the heart.[50, 51] If epinephrine was included in the local anesthetic mixture, however, significant systemic effects of the adrenergic drug, including tachycardia and decreased arterial pressure, could be seen.[51]

MYOCARDIAL PERFUSION AND OXYGENATION

Coronary blood flow has been and is still difficult and cumbersome to measure, even in animals. In addition, documentation of blood flow and oxygen consumption does not indicate the adequacy of myocardial perfusion and oxygenation. This is true partly because the predominant control of coronary blood flow is through alterations in coronary vascular resistance induced by changes in cardiac oxygenation. The subject of control of coronary circulation and indices of myocardial oxygenation is beyond the scope of this review. In general, if an intact heart is using lactate, it is reasonably well oxygenated.[52]

There has been much less investigation of the effect of anesthetics on coronary blood flow and oxygen supply to the heart than that previously described for ventricular function. It is of some interest that the earliest published study was in man, in which a 50 percent decrease in both arterial pressure and coronary blood flow was demonstrated after spinal anesthesia.[53] Calculated cardiac work fell to the same extent as coronary blood flow, with no changes in oxygen or lactate extraction; consequently, the investigators concluded that the fall in coronary blood flow was in response to decreased oxygen demand of the heart. Published studies in both animal and man since that investigation have generally come to the same conclusion with other anesthetics. The most complete results have been from a multidepartmental team in Gottingen, West Germany, which has reported the effects of a number of intravenous drugs, including ketamine,[44] droperidol-fentanyl,[44] and thiopental,[36] on myocardial blood flow and metabolism in man. Recently, we have also investigated halothane. In general, changes in coronary blood flow and oxygen consumption paralleled changes in the determinants of myocardial oxygen demand, namely heart rate, systemic blood pressure, and the contractile function of the heart. There have been animal studies that suggest some inhalation anesthetics may directly affect coronary vascular resistance,[54-56] but these results have been conflicting. It seems very likely that the coronary vascular muscle can be dilated by potent negative inotropic drugs. However, the bulk of the evidence at present is that in intact animals and man, the effect of anesthetics on coronary blood flow is directly related to the myocardial oxygen supply-demand relationship.[29, 57] When myocardial oxygen demand is increased, so is coronary blood flow; when myocardial oxygen demand is decreased, coronary blood flow also decreases.

CLINICAL IMPLICATIONS

All the results that have been described thus far have been in healthy volunteers or patients. The patients that the clinician is most often concerned about are those with diseased hearts. Within the last five years, there have been a number of investigations that have looked at anesthetic effects in patients with diseased hearts. In some instances, they have shown very similar effects. In general, the narcotic analgesics produced minimal effects on ventricular function in patients with ischemic and valvular heart disease.[41, 58, 59] Although diazepam also appears to produce minimal changes in ventricular function in patients with heart disease, one study of patients with ischemic heart disease did document a decrease in stroke volume after 0.12 mg/kg.[60] However, there was also a slight decrease in preload at the same time. Stoelting and Gibbs have shown that the addition of nitrous oxide to morphine in patients with both valvular heart disease and ischemic heart disease resulted in a 20 to 25 percent decrease in stroke volume.[61] The same was not true with the combination of fentanyl and droperidol. Low concentrations of halothane did not appear to be deleterious to patients with ischemic heart disease.[58, 62] In fact, recent studies suggest that perhaps low concentrations of halothane may actually be beneficial to the oxygen supply-demand ratio in patients with ischemic heart disease.[63] Of considerable theoretic interest was the demonstration by Wiberg-Jorgensen, Skovsted, and Misfeldt[64] that low concentrations of fluroxene (which resulted in no change at all in cardiovascular dynamics in healthy patients[13]) severely depressed stroke volume in patients with aortic valvular disease. Low concentrations of isoflurane produced more decrease in stroke volume and arterial blood pressure in patients with ischemic heart disease than had been seen in healthy patients.[62]

In conclusion, then, one cannot draw firm results from studies of the effect of anesthetics on cardiac function in healthy individuals and transpose them to patients with heart disease. This observer believes that the only way to safely anesthetize such patients is to titrate the anesthetic (whatever it may be) against the best measure of ventricular function available. As our monitoring techniques become more and more sophisticated, this approach becomes more valid. Knowledge of the effect of these drugs on the normal individual allows an educated approach to their use in patients with heart disease.

REFERENCES

1. Flacke, W., and Alper, M. H.: *Actions of halothane and norepinephrine in isolated mammalian heart.* Anesthesiology 23:793, 1962.
2. Price, H.L.: *Circulatory actions of general anesthetic agents and the*

homeostatic roles of epinephrine and norepinephrine in man. Clin. Pharmacol. 2:163, 1961.

3. Shepherd, J.T.: *Interthoracic baroreflexes.* Mayo Clin. Proc. 48:426, 1973.

4. Siegel, J.H.: *The myocardial contractile state and its role in response to anesthesia and surgery.* Anesthesiology 30:519, 1969.

5. Shimosato, S., and Etsten, B.E.: *Effect of anesthetic drugs on the heart; a critical review of myocardial contractility and its relation to hemodynamics.* Clin. Anesth. 3:17, 1969.

6. Merin, R.G.: *Effect of anesthetics on the heart.* Surg. Clin. North Am. 55:759, 1975.

7. Humphrey, C.B., Oury, J.H., Virgilio, R.W., et al.: *An analysis of direct and indirect measurements of left atrial filling pressure.* J. Thor. Cardiovasc. Surg. 71:643, 1976.

8. Prys-Roberts, C., Gersh, B.J., Baker, A.B., et al.: *Effects of halothane on the interactions between myocardial contractility, aortic impedance and left ventricular performance. I. Theoretical considerations and results.* Br. J. Anaesth. 44:634, 1972.

9. Sarnoff, S.T.: *Myocardial contractility as described by ventricular function curves.* Physiol. Rev. 35:107, 1955.

10. Skovsted, P., and Price, H.L.: *Effects of ethrane on arterial pressure, preganglionic sympathetic activity and barostatic reflexes.* Anesthesiology 36:257, 1972.

11. Jones, R.E., Linde, H.W., Deutsch, S., et al.: *Hemodynamic actions of diethyl ether in normal man.* Anesthesiology 23:299, 1962.

12. Gregory, G.A., Eger, E.I., Smith, N.T., et al.: *Cardiovascular effects of diethyl ether in man.* Anesthesiology 34:19, 1971.

13. Cullen, B.F., Eger, E.I., Smith, N.T., et al.: *Cardiovascular effects of fluroxene in man.* Anesthesiology 32:218, 1970.

14. Etsten, B.E., Reynolds, R.N., and Li, T.H.: *Effects of controlled respiration on circulation during cyclopropane anesthesia.* Anesthesiology 16:365, 1955.

15. Cullen, D.J., Eger, E.I., Gregory, G.A., et al.: *Cardiovascular effects of cyclopropane in man.* Anesthesiology 31:398, 1969.

16. Price, H.L., Skovsted, P., Pauca, A.L., et al.: *Evidence for beta-receptor activation produced by halothane in normal man.* Anesthesiology 32:389, 1970.

17. Eger, E.I., Smith, N.T., Stoelting, R.K., et al.: *Cardiovascular effects of halothane in man.* Anesthesiology 32:396, 1970.

18. Filner, B.E., and Karliner, J.H.: *Alterations of normal left ventricular performance by general anesthesia.* Anesthesiology 45:610, 1976.

19. Libonati, M., Cooperman, L.H., and Price, H.L.: *Time dependent circulatory effects of methoxyflurane in man.* Anesthesiology 34:439, 1971.

20. Levesque, P.R., Nanagas, V., Shanks, C., et al.: *Circulatory effects of enflurane in normocarbic human volunteers.* Can. Anaesth. Soc. J. 21:580, 1974.

21. Haldemann, G., Schmid, E., Frey, P., et al.: *Wirkung von Ethrane auf die Kreislaufgrossen Geriatrischer Patienten.* der Anaesthetist 24:343, 1975.

22. Stevens, W.C., Cromwell, T.H., Halsey, M.H., et al.: *Cardiovascular effects of a new inhalation anesthetic, Forane, in human volunteers at constant arterial carbon dioxide tension.* Anesthesiology 35:8, 1971.

23. Katz, R.L., and Bigger, J.T.: *Cardiac arrhythmias during anesthesia and operation.* Anesthesiology 33:193, 1970.

24. Jorfeldt, L., Lofstrom, B., Miller, J., et al.: *Propranolol in ether anesthesia.* Acta Anaesthesiol. Scand. 11:159, 1967.

25. Price, H.L., Jones, R.E., Deutsch, S., et al.: *Ventricular function and autonomic nervous activity during cyclopropane anesthesia in man.* J. Clin. Invest. 41:604, 1962.

26. Mahaffey, J.C., Aldinger, E.E., Sprouse, J.H., et al.: *The cardiovascular effects of halothane.* Anesthesiology 22:952, 1961.

27. Sonntag, H., Donath, U., Hillebrand, W., et al.: *Left ventricular function in conscious humans and during halothane anesthesia.* Anesthesiology, 1978, in press.

28. Graves, C.L., and Downs, N.H.: *Cardiovascular and renal effects of enflurane in surgical patients.* Anesth. Analg. (Cleve.) 53:898, 1974.

29. Merin, R.G., Kumazawa, T., and Luka, N.L.: *Enflurane depresses myocardial function, perfusion and metabolism in the dog.* Anesthesiology 45:501, 1976.

30. Calverley, R.K., Smith, N.T., Prys-Roberts, C., et al.: *Cardiovascular effects of enflurane anesthesia during controlled ventilation in man.* Anesthesiology, 1978, in press.

31. Eisele, J.H., and Smith, N.T.: *Cardiovascular effects of 40 per cent nitrous oxide in man.* Anesth. Analg. (Cleve.) 51:956, 1972.

32. Wong, K.C., Martin, W.E., Hornbein, T.F., et al.: *Cardiovascular effects of morphine sulphate with oxygen and nitrous oxide in man.* Anesthesiology 38:542, 1973.

33. Smith, N.T., Eger, E.I., Stoelting, R.K., et al.: *The cardiovascular and sympathomimetic responses to the addition of nitrous oxide to halothane in man.* Anesthesiology 32:410, 1970.

34. Smith, N.T., Eger, E.I., Gregory, G.A., et al.: *The cardiovascular responses to the addition of nitrous oxide to diethyl ether in man.* Can. Anaesth. Soc. J. 19:42, 1972.

35. Etsten, B.E., and Li, T.H.: *Hemodynamic changes during thiopental anesthesia in humans: cardiac output, stroke volume, tidal peripheral resistance and intrathoracic blood volume.* J. Clin. Invest. 34:500, 1955.

36. Sonntag, H., Helberg, K., Shenk, H.D., et al.: *Effects of thiopental on coronary blood flow and myocardial metabolism in man.* Acta Anaesthesiol. Scand. 19:69, 1975.

37. Rao, S., Sherbanink, R.W., Prasad, K., et al.: *Cardiopulmonary effects of diazepam.* Clin. Pharmacol. 14:182, 1973.

38. Schenk, H.D., Sonntag, H., Kettler, D., et al.: *Der Einfluss von Epontol auf den Sauerstoffverbrauch des Herzens und die Haemodynamik beim Menschen.* Der Anaesthetist 23:105, 1974.

39. Sonntag, H., Heiss, H.W., Regensberger, D., et al.: *Effects of althesin on coronary blood flow and myocardial metabolism in man.* Acta Anaesthesiol. Scand. 17:218, 1973.

40. Kettler, D., Sonntag, H., Donath, U., et al.: *Haemodynamik, Myokardmechanik, Sauerstoffbedarf und Sauerstoffversorgung des menschlichen Herzens unter Narkoseeinleutung mit Etomidate.* Der Anaesthetist 23:116, 1974.

41. Lowenstein, E., Hallowell, P., Levine, F.L., et al.: *Cardiovascular responses to large doses of intravenous morphine in man.* N. Engl. J. Med. 281:1389, 1969.

42. Graves, C.L., Downs, N.H., and Browne, A.B.: *Cardiovascular effects of minimal analgesic quantities of Innovar, fentanyl and droperidol in man.* Anesth. Analg. (Cleve.) 54:15, 1975.

43. Tweed, W.A., and Mymin, D.: *Myocardial force-velocity relationship during ketamine anesthesia at constant heart rate.* Anesthesiology 41:49, 1974.

44. Sonntag, H., Heiss, H.W., Regensberger, D., et al.: *Koronare Haemodynamik unter Narkose-einleitung mit Dehydrobenzperidol/Fentanyl und Ketamine.* Langenbecks Archiv. Klin. Chir. (Suppl. Chirurg. Forum) p. 301, 1972.

45. Ferrari, H.A., Borten, F.J., Talton, I.H., et al.: *Action of droperidol and fentanyl on cardiac output and related hemodynamic parameters.* South. Med. J. 67:49, 1974.

46. Longnecker, D.E., Stoelting, R.K., and Morrow, A.G.: *Cardiac and peripheral vascular effects of d-tubocurare in man.* Anesth. Analg. (Cleve.) 49:660, 1970.

47. Longnecker, D.E., Stoelting, R.K., and Morrow, A.G.: *Cardiac and peripheral vascular effects of gallamine in man.* Anesth. Analg. (Cleve.) 52:935, 1973.

48. Stoelting, R.K.: *Hemodynamic effects of pancuronium and d-tubocurare in anesthetized patients.* Anesthesiology 36:612, 1972.

49. Cooperman, L.H.: *Succinylcholine induced hyperkalemia in neuromuscular disease.* J.A.M.A. 213:1867, 1970.

59. Shimosato, S., and Etsten, B.E.: *Role of the venous system in cardiocirculatory dynamics during spinal and epidural anesthesia in man.* Anesthesiology 30:619, 1969.

51. Bonica, J.J., Akamatsu, T.J., Berges, P.V., et al.: *Circulatory effects*

EFFECTS OF ANESTHETICS ON THE HEART

of peridural block. II. Effects of epinephrine. Anesthesiology 34:514, 1971.

52. Merin, R.G.: *Inhalation anesthetics and myocardial metabolism.* Anesthesiology 39:216, 1973.
53. Hackel, D.B., Sancetta, S.M., and Kleinerman, J.: *Effect of hypotension due to spinal anesthesia on coronary blood flow and myocardial metabolism in man.* Circulation 13:92, 1956.
54 Wolff, G., Claudi, B., Rist, M., et al.: *Regulation of coronary blood flow during ether and halothane anesthesia.* Br. J. Anaesth. 44:1139, 1972.
55. Vatner, S.F., and Smith, N.T.: *Effects of halothane on left ventricular function and distribution of regional blood flow in dogs and primates.* Circ. Res. 34:155, 1974.
56. Domenech, R. J., Macho, P., Valdez, J., et al.: *Coronary vascular resistance during halothane anesthesia.* Anesthesiology 46:236, 1977.
57. Merin, R.G., Kumazawa, T., and Luka, N.L.: *Myocardial function and metabolism in the conscious dog and during halothane anesthesia.* Anesthesiology 44:402, 1976.
58. Stoelting, R.K., Creaser, C.W., Gibbs, P.S., et al.: *Circulatory effects of halothane added to morphine anesthesia in patients with coronary artery disease.* Anesth. Analg. (Cleve.) 53:449, 1974.
59. Stoelting, R.K., Gibbs, P.S., Creaser, C.W., et al.: *Hemodynamic and ventilatory responses to fentanyl, fentanyl-droperidol, and nitrous oxide in patients with acquired valvular heart disease.* Anesthesiology 42:319, 1975.
60. Cote, P., Gueret, P., and Bourassa, M.: *Systemic and coronary hemodynamic effects of diazepam in patients with normal and diseased coronary arteries.* Circulation 50:1210, 1974.
61. Stoelting, R.K., and Gibbs, P.S.: *Hemodynamic effects of morphine and morphine-nitrous oxide in valvular heart disease and coronary artery disease.* Anesthesiology 38:45, 1973.
62. Mallow, J.E., White, R.P., Cucchiara, R.F., et al.: *Hemodynamic effects of isoflurane and halothane in patients with coronary artery disease.* Anesth. Analg. (Cleve.) 55:135, 1976.
63. Kistner, J.R., Miller, E.D., Lake, C.L., et al.: *Indices of myocardial oxygenation during coronary revascularization in man with morphine vs. halothane anesthesia.* Anesthesiology, 1978, in press.
64. Wiberg-Jorgensen, F., Skovsted, P., and Misfeldt, B.: *Cardiovascular hemodynamics in patients with aortic valvular disease.* Acta Anaesthesiol. Scand. 17:136, 1973.

MONITORING THE CARDIOVASCULAR SYSTEM DURING ANESTHESIA

Casey D. Blitt, M.D.

Dr. Blitt explores two areas: the present state of the art of monitoring the cardiovascular system, and methods of both invasive and noninvasive monitoring. Included is the use of the external jugular J-wire technique developed by Dr. Blitt.

Burnell R. Brown, Jr.

According to *Webster's Dictionary,* the definition of a monitor is "that which warns, advises, or cautions." All anesthetic agents and techniques affect the cardiovascular system either in a major or minor manner, and this is especially important for the patient with pre-existing heart disease. It is the anesthesiologist's job, using his skill and past experience, to insure that the patient's life is not threatened by the cardiovascular effects of anesthetics. Many anesthetics have been successfully administered without any monitor other than a finger on the pulse and observation of the color of the patient's skin. Recent advances in instrumentation and technology make it possible, however, for the anesthesiologist to obtain valuable information regarding the patient's cardiovascular system, and these new advances should be employed whenever possible. Necessary information must be obtained so that the anesthesiologist can be reasonably certain of the cardiovascular status of the patient. The information must be assimilated by the anesthesiologist, in the context of both time and complexity, allowing him to make decisions, act on these decisions, and detect trends that may be deleterious to the patient. Accepting this precept, then, the question that arises is: What should be monitored and when and how does the anesthesiologist go about utilizing available monitoring techniques?

The anesthesiologist needs to know if the cardiovascular system is functioning properly and if the needs of the patient's vital organs are being supplied or something is in jeopardy. Variables of the cardiovascular system that may supply valuable data in this regard include (1) the electrical activity of the heart, (2) the effectiveness of the heart as a pump, (3) the state of the peripheral circulation, and (4) information from various organs that reflect adequacy of perfusion.

Information regarding these variables can be obtained invasively and noninvasively and continuously or intermittently. I will discuss many types of monitors and combinations of methods to provide the best cardiovascular data for each individual patient.

ELECTRICAL ACTIVITY OF THE HEART

The surface electrocardiogram (ECG) is a valuable monitor in the operating room. It is important to emphasize that the beat-to-beat oscilloscopic display of the ECG is different than the diagnostic 12-lead ECG, and I intend to discuss the uses of the ECG intraoperatively and in the recovery room. It must always be remembered that the ECG is not a measure of the heart as a pump, but is primarily a measure of electrical activity. The ECG can indicate

1. the presence and continuity of the electrical activity of the heart;
2. the cardiac rhythm;
3. the ST segment changes that warn of myocardial ischemia or injury;
4. the changes in depolarization and repolarization of the atria and ventricles, such as those that occur in electrolyte disturbances;
5. the heart rate (under usual circumstances);
6. the baseline for the timing of mechanical cardiac events.

A good signal is important in determining the anesthesiologist's ability to interpret a given electrocardiographic signal. Despite many recent advances in the technology of physiologic monitors, none is capable of functioning properly in the presence of an active electrocautery unit. Lead II is most commonly used intraoperatively. This lead is parallel to the P wave vector and makes the P wave easy to identify, especially when the observer is trying to differentiate ventricular from supraventricular arrhythmias. A good oscilloscopic trace of the ECG on lead II is invaluable intraoperatively and should be used routinely in patients with any sort of pre-existing heart disease. The presence or absence of the P wave is especially important in enabling the anesthesiologist to determine the hemodynamic effect of the "atrial kick." Synchronous contraction of the atria provides an important assistance in ventricular filling and is associated with a better cardiac output than when no P waves are present.

In patients with heart disease, an indication of myocardial ischemia should be the goal of electrocardiographic monitoring. It is difficult to determine in which patients myocardial oxygen supply will not be able to keep pace with demand. Patients with hypertension, cardiomyopathies, generalized arteriosclerotic vascular disease, coronary artery disease, and valvular heart disease should all be suspect for myocardial ischemia. For this purpose, the limb leads are inadequate. A lead is needed that looks at the area of the precordium most susceptible to ischemia, namely, that area supplied by the left anterior descending coronary artery. It has been shown that 89 percent of ST segment information obtained in the conventional 12-lead ECG is found in lead V_5. I recommend that a V_5 lead be routinely monitored in patients with heart disease. In patients with coronary artery disease, even more leads should be monitored, but at least a combination of V_5 and lead II should be routinely performed.

How is this accomplished? If your monitor has 5-lead capability, there is no problem. Merely connect the four limb electrodes in the normal position and place the fifth electrode in the V_5 position (fifth intercostal space at the anterior axillary line). If you have a 3-lead monitor, (1) place the left arm lead in the fifth intercostal space at the anterior axillary line, (2) place the right arm lead on the right shoulder, and (3) place the third lead on the left shoulder. Set the physiological monitor selection switch to AVF, if it exists on lead II (Fig. 1). This will enable you to look at the anterior surface of the left ventricle. Horizontal or downsloping ST segment depression greater than 1 mm or any ST elevation suggests myocardial ischemia. Early detection of such ischemia should then allow the anesthesiologist to take appropriate therapeutic intervention to reduce myocardial oxygen demand.

It may be necessary to protect the V_5 lead from the operative site or from being washed off by surgical preparation solution.

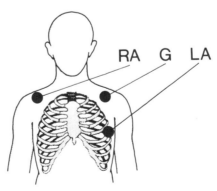

Figure 1. Placement of leads in 3-lead monitor. LA = left arm lead; RA = right arm lead; G = third lead.

This can be accomplished by placing a small Steridrape® over the lead to protect it, to keep it out of the surgical field, and to keep it dry. Only operations on the left anterior chest will require alternate lead placement. The aim of this alternate placement should be to obtain as close an approximation to a V_5 lead as possible.

His's bundle electrocardiography can also be used to facilitate recognition of certain conduction disturbances by more precisely defining the PR interval. An esophageal lead can also be used, especially in cases in which P waves are difficult to evaluate. The instrumentation and techniques involved in obtaining information from these two modalities are invasive (as compared with the noninvasive surface ECG) and somewhat complex. They are beyond the scope of our discussion.

THE HEART AS A PUMP

Assessment of the heart as a pump involves a complex interaction of mechanical myocardial performance, myocardial contractility, and blood pressure. Information regarding these variables may be obtained invasively or noninvasively. The monitoring modalities that may be employed in any particular patient depend on the severity of the patient's cardiovascular disease, the technical expertise and ability of the anesthesiologist involved, and the availability of equipment to carry out the monitoring techniques.

Mechanical Performance

Mechanical performance is essentially an assessment of the heart's ability to eject blood against a peripheral load. Cardiac output is the *sine qua non* of myocardial performance. Cardiac performance involves complex interactions of a number of factors, including end-diastolic fiber length, peripheral resistance, heart rate, and myocardial contractile state. Noninvasive methods of determining myocardial performance include:
   1. precordial or esophageal stethoscopy
   2. use of the Doppler ultrasonic flow meter
   3. measurement of systolic time intervals
   4. pneumocardiography

5. impedance cardiography
6. echocardiography
7. nuclear cardiology

Of all these monitoring devices, the precordial or esophageal stethoscope is the easiest to implement and provides the anesthesiologist with continuous information regarding mechanical performance of the heart. A change in the quality or character of the heart sounds is easily detected using this technique and serves as an early warning to the anesthesiologist of potential impending problems. This monitor should be routinely used in all patients, including those with any degree of cardiovascular disease.

The Doppler ultrasonic flow meter is a modification of Doppler technology. New prototype devices are capable of providing a noninvasive assessment of stroke volume and ventricular function, utilizing a probe placed on the suprasternal notch. Probes are also being developed to assess ventricular function using measurement of flow acceleration with the probe placed on the patient's wrist. Certain computer techniques and advances are necessary to automatically adjust the probe and to perform the complex calculations necessary; therefore, this technique cannot be currently used.

Systolic time intervals, pneumocardiography, and impedance cardiography are frought with many technical problems that must be solved before they become useful clinical modalities. Farther in the future the echocardiogram and nuclear cardiology represent real potential for noninvasive measurement of cardiac function. These two methods are capable of detecting myocardial ischemia and ejection fraction noninvasively. The technology necessary to utilize these two methods has not yet progressed far enough to enable their use in the operating room.

At this point in time, then, precise measurement of cardiac performance must rely upon invasive techniques. I will discuss two invasive monitors for determination of mechanical myocardial performance: central venous system cannulation and pulmonary artery cannulation.

Although frequently maligned, measurement of central venous pressure (CVP) remains a useful technique in the operating room. It is considerably easier to implement than measurement of pulmonary artery pressure. If used carefully and with wisdom, measurement of central venous pressure can often yield valuable information, somewhat similar to that of pulmonary artery pressure. It must be remembered, however, that CVP reflects the right side of the circulation and not the left. Even in patients with cardiac disease, CVP can be used to assess the adequacy of a patient's vascular volume and, very indirectly, the adequacy of ventricular filling. CVP may not be reliable, however, in patients with severe left ventricular disease.

Any cause of increased intrathoracic pressure, such as positive pressure ventilation, pneumothorax, abdominal distention, or cardiac tamponade, can increase the CVP. There are many occasions in which CVP can be normal and the pulmonary artery wedge pressure significantly elevated. It is also possible for the CVP to be elevated and the pulmonary artery pressure normal. Proper interpretation of CVP requires a working knowledge of cardiac physiology.

An interesting anecdote of the value of CVP was reported to me recently. A patient who had undergone a four-vessel coronary artery bypass operation had successfully emerged from cardiopulmonary bypass, and all was apparently well. Central venous pressure and pulmonary capillary wedge pressure were both being monitored. Although the wedge pressure remained normal, the CVP continued to rise inexplicably. Even though no apparent reason for the rise in CVP could be found, the surgeon was asked to examine his grafts. On examination it was found that the graft to the right coronary artery was nonfunctional and completely occluded, resulting in acute right ventricular failure. The CVP was a definite aid in this diagnosis.

Recent literature and clinical experience would suggest that the jugular veins, external or internal, represent the easiest, most reliable method of obtaining access to the central circulation. Cannulation of these veins should be performed in the Trendelenburg position. The right side of the neck is preferable because of the proximity to the superior vena cava. The internal jugular vein should be cannulated at approximately the medial border of the clavicular head of the sternocleidodomastoid muscle. It lies just lateral to the carotid artery at this point. A small gauge (22 gauge) needle should be used to locate the vein prior to cannulation with a larger catheter. All cannulations of the internal jugular vein should be performed using sterile technique, when possible.

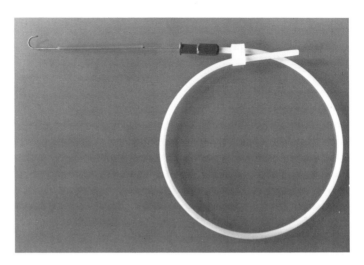

Figure 2. J-wire.

The external jugular vein is accessible to the anesthesiologist and is an excellent access to the central venous system. A method has been developed that uses a flexible angiographic wire catheter guide or J-wire* (Fig. 2) to aid in passing the catheter into the superior vena cava. This technique overcomes problems encountered owing to acute angulation of the vein or difficulty passing the catheters through the venous valves and has proven to be dependable and safe (Fig. 3). After sterile preparation, the external jugular vein is cannulated with a short, over-the-needle Teflon placement unit. After successful placement of the catheter in the external vein, the J-wire is threaded through this initial catheter until it is estimated to be well into the thorax. The initial catheter is then removed and a definitive catheter (6 to 7 in. long) is passed over the wire guide and into the superior vena cava. The J-wire is then removed.

This technique represents a significant advance in regard to complications, and I highly recommend it to the practitioner who may be fearful of the complications of subclavian or internal jugular vein cannulation. A comparison of various CVP methods is seen in Table 1.

Because mechanical performance is dependent on a number

*Argon Medical Products, Inc., Garland, Texas.

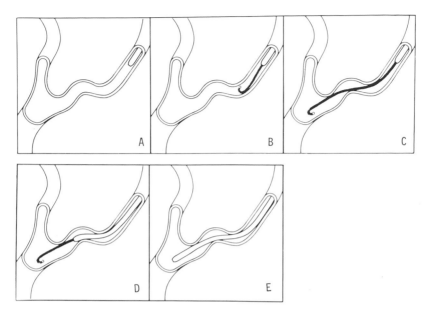

Figure 3. The J-wire technique for passing a catheter into the superior vena cava. *A,* Catheter placed in vein. *B,* J-wire advances past first obstruction. *C,* J-wire is completely inserted. *D,* Catheter advances over J-wire. *E,* Catheter is completely advanced and the J-wire is removed.

of variables, its measurement has long been a thorn in the side of the anesthesiologist, especially in the operating room. Currently, the best measure of cardiac performance is cardiac output. Passage of a catheter into the pulmonary artery enables the determination of cardiac output using the thermodilution technique. Additionally, true mixed venous blood may be obtained for calculation of intrapulmonary shunting. Pulmonary capillary wedge pressure or pulmonary artery occluded pressure provides an indirect measure of left atrial pressure, which helps us estimate left ventricular filling pressure. The combination of arterial pressure, pulmonary capillary wedge pressure, and cardiac output can produce extremely useful information. Pulmonary artery catheterization is quite invasive, and the value of obtainable information must be weighed against the risk to the patient. Patients with heart disease who are undergoing cardiac surgery, major vascular surgery, major intra-abdominal surgery,

Table 1. Advantages of Various CVP Methods.

	Technique			
	External Jugular	Internal Jugular	Subclavian	Brachial
Simplicity & ease of insertion	+ +	+	–	+
Success rate	+ +	+ +	+ +	– –
Complications	+ +	0	– –	+
Long-term adaptability	–	–	+ +	0
Accessibility during anesthesia	+ +	+ +	–	–
Ability to insert PA catheter	+	+ +	0	–

+ Advantage, – Disadvantage, 0 Not a factor

and major neurological procedures are all good candidates for pulmonary artery catheterization.

Use of a pulmonary artery catheter requires a fair amount of instrumentation, such as a pressure transducer and oscilloscopic display for measurement (for section on radial artery catheterization), a continuous heparinized flush apparatus, and a computer for measuring cardiac output. The thermodilution method for determining cardiac output has achieved great popularity because it is inexpensive (saline is extremely cheap), but it does have some inherent errors. This means that, regardless of the numbers obtained using a cardiac output computer, the numbers must be examined with the patient's clinical status in mind. For determining cardiac output, a special pulmonary artery catheter must be used, which contains a thermister located at or slightly behind the tip of the balloon. This catheter has an additional lumen for injection of cold saline into the right atrium, and the thermister measures the change of temperature in the pulmonary artery.

Newer monitoring devices are currently being produced that will allow a beat-to-beat determination of cardiac output following calibration of the instrument with a cardiac output determined by thermodilution. Pulmonary artery catheters are best inserted via the internal jugular vein, although the external jugular vein using the J-wire technique can be employed. Insertion of a pulmonary artery catheter requires a large introducer sheath aided by a dilator. During passage of the flow-directed pulmonary artery catheter, proper placement must be verified by identification of the appropriate pressure traces on an oscilloscope (Fig. 4). Simultaneous display of the ECG is recommended. The length of the catheter is marked in 10 cm intervals. Using the right internal jugular vein, the right atrium is encountered at 25 to 35 cm, the right ventricle at 35 to 45 cm, and the pulmonary artery at 45 to 55 cm. The catheter should be advanced in the pulmonary artery until the wedge tracing is observed, and deflation of the balloon should restore the pulmonary artery trace. The balloon should remain inflated while the catheter is advanced, until wedge pressure is obtained. Withdrawal of the catheter should only be performed with the balloon *deflated.* Once the catheter is in satisfactory position, the balloon should remain deflated except when actual wedge pressures are being taken. One must be alert for development of a "permanent wedge" position caused by the catheter, with balloon deflated, creeping out of the pulmonary artery. If a wedge pressure is observed while the balloon is deflated, the catheter should be pulled back until the pulmonary artery trace reappears.

For proper assessment of the pharmacologic and physiologic actions of various cardiotonic and vasoactive agents in cardiac patients, measurement of pulmonary capillary wedge pressure and cardiac output is almost mandatory.

The most significant concepts that have resulted from the use of the pulmonary artery catheter are those regarding changes in cardiac performance that occur during anesthesia because of failure of the left ventricle. The left ventricular muscle is usually depressed by the use of anesthetic agents and can fail to eject

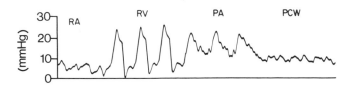

Figure 4. Pressure traces on an oscilloscope. The Y-axis indicates normal pressure ranges in various chambers of the heart and pulmonary vasculature. RA = right atrium; RV = right ventricle; PA = pulmonary artery; PCW = pulmonary capillary wedge.

blood against increased peripheral loads or increased resistance to blood flow. This concept, namely, that the failing ventricle does not *fail to fill* but *fails to empty,* has been highlighted by the use of a pulmonary catheter. Along these same lines, the performance of a failing left ventricle under an increased afterload can be improved by *reducing* the afterload using vasodilator drugs, rather than by "flogging" the heart with inotropic agents.

Myocardial Contractility

Many factors affect contractility. Contractility is a complex relationship between time, force developed in the heart muscle, fiber length, and velocity of shortening. Indeed, contractility is difficult to define and can probably best be described as "oomph." The best accepted measurement of contractility is left ventricular dP/dt. Unfortunately, this measurement requires that a catheter be passed retrograde into the left ventricle, and consequently this technique is not particularly well suited to routine monitoring.

Blood Pressure

Blood pressure has always been considered an important measurement during the conduct of an anesthetic. The cardiovascular system is designed to maintain systemic arterial pressure within a tightly constrained range. The baroreceptor reflexes, indeed, depend upon intravascular sensors, which detect changes in blood pressure. Noninvasive techniques for measuring blood pressure include sphygmomanometry, ultrasonic Doppler detection, plethysmograph flow detection, and oscillotonometry.

The use of the occluding cuff (sphygmomanometry) is the most widely employed method for measuring systemic arterial pressure. The sounds of Korotkoff are well known to all practicing anesthesiologists. The values for systolic and diastolic arterial pressures obtained in man using this technique have been shown to correlate fairly well with values obtained by direct intra-arterial methods. At the higher and lower ranges of pressures, however, Korotkoff's sounds may be inaccurate. These indirect measurements underestimate true arterial pressure at values above 160 torr and tend to overestimate pressures below 100 torr. This occurs despite rigorous attention to details, such as the width of the cuff, its placement, and the rate of deflation, as well as the precise location of the stethoscope over the artery. Nevertheless, the use of the blood pressure cuff continues to be our first-line monitor for arterial pressure.

The Doppler apparatus has been shown to be more accurate than Korotkoff's sounds and has enjoyed considerable popularity in recent years. Its primary advantages exist in those situations in which Korotkoff's sounds are difficult to obtain and in pediatric patients. This method requires instrumentation incorporating an oscillator, a detector, and an amplifier circuit.

Direct measurement of arterial pressure via cannulation of a peripheral artery is becoming extremely popular as anesthesiologists increasingly realize the value of continuous measurements, which can detect rapid changes in a patient's condition. This type of beat-to-beat monitoring of arterial pressure is useful in open-heart procedures, deliberate hypotensive anesthesia, open-chest procedures, major vascular procedures, and neurosurgical procedures, as well as in patients with moderate to severe cardiovascular disease. The continuous nature of the information provided, as well as the ability to sample blood frequently for determination of blood gas, makes arterial catheterization a technique that should be part of every anesthesiologist's armamentarium. Vessels that can be used for cannulation include the radial, ulnar, dorsalis pedis, brachial, axillary, superficial temporal, and femoral arteries. The radial artery is most easily cannulated with few major problems and thus should be the artery of first choice.

Prior to cannulation of the radial artery, an Allen's test should be performed to ascertain adequacy of ulnar collateral flow. It is important to determine if ulnar flow is sufficient to supply blood to the hand if the radial artery should become occluded. In the Allen's test, both the radial and ulnar arteries are occluded by the examiner and the patient is instructed to alternately clench and open his hand several times. The hand is then opened and seen to be blanched. Pressure over only the ulnar artery is then released, and if ulnar collateral circulation is adequate, the color of the hand will return to normal (blush) within a few seconds. I recommend that a radial artery not be cannulated if circulation does not seem to be restored within 15 seconds. It is important that the hand not be completely extended when the test is performed, because complete extension of the hand with wide extension of the fingers can occlude the transpalmar arch, and this will result in parts of the finger and palm remaining blanched indefinitely, thereby giving rise to a false positive test.

Small gauge (20 or 22 gauge), nontapered, nonradiopaque Teflon catheters should be used because these catheters have been associated with the lowest incidences of arterial thrombosis and occlusion.

If the radial artery is not available or if the Allen's test indicates that the radial artery should not be cannulated, the dorsalis pedis, brachial, or axillary arteries represent viable alternatives. Indeed, the continuous use of on-line monitoring devices, currently available to measure continuously arterial carbon dioxide and oxygen tensions, requires a large-caliber vessel such as the brachial or axillary arteries.

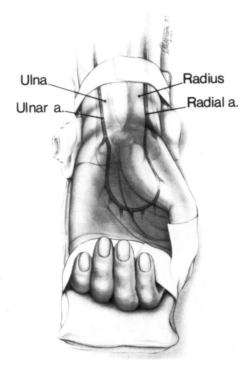

Figure 5. Wrist dorsiflexed for percutaneous radial artery cannulation.

Percutaneous radial artery cannulation should be performed with the wrist dorsiflexed to about a 50- or 60-degree angle (Fig. 5). The supinated hand and forearm should be fixed to an arm board and the wrist dorsiflexed over a towel or gauze sponges. The catheter is inserted along the course of the radial artery at approximately a 15- to 20-degree angle to the surface of the skin. A free spurt of bright red blood indicates entry into the vessel, and at this point the needle is held fixed and the cannula advanced into the arterial lumen. The needle is then withdrawn and the cannula connected to nondistensible tubing, a continuous flush apparatus, and a strain gauge-oscilloscope for display purposes.

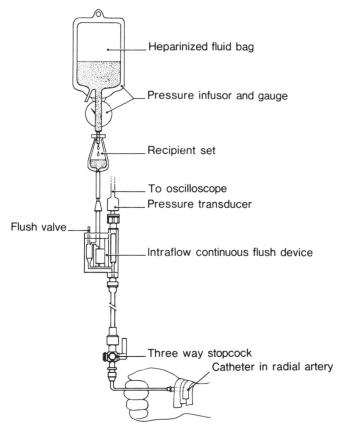

Figure 6. Flush apparatus for catheter.

The catheter must be flushed continuously with a heparin solution containing 1 to 2 units/ml heparin in physiologic saline solution at a rate of 1.5 to 3 ml/hr. This is important in minimizing thrombosis formation, keeping the wave-form from becoming excessively dampened, and preventing cerebral embolization from flushing with too large a volume of solution. Forceful flushing with a large volume of solution in excess of 2.5 ml should be avoided. A schematic diagram of the flush apparatus is seen in Figure 6.

The primary complications of arterial cannulation are related to thrombosis and occlusion of the vessel. A test for adequate collateral circulation can obviate these problems.

STATE OF THE PERIPHERAL CIRCULATION

The true state of the peripheral circulation can be assessed by calculating total peripheral resistance. Calculation of this information requires determination of cardiac output and consequently can only be adequately assessed in patients in whom cardiac output is already being determined.

OTHER ORGANS AND MONITORS REFLECTING ADEQUACY OF PERFUSION

Probably the single most important additional piece of information that can be obtained in patients with heart disease is adequacy of urine output, which indicates satisfactory renal perfusion. In patients with moderate or severe cardiac disease, especially those undergoing major surgical operations, an indwelling urinary catheter can provide extremely valuable information.

The cardiovascular system is dependent upon temperature, and, consequently, it is my feeling that temperature should be monitored in all patients with cardiovascular disease who are undergoing surgery. Arterial oxygen tension is also important in patients with cardiac disease because it is important to ensure that the myocardium is potentially being exposed to an adequate oxygen tension. This measurement is easy to perform in patients with an indwelling arterial catheter. In patients in whom an indwelling arterial catheter is not used, intermittent arterial blood samples can provide valuable information regarding the degree of arterial oxygenation.

I would now like to provide a guide for what I consider to be appropriate monitoring for patients with varying degrees of cardiovascular disease who are undergoing anesthesia and surgery.

Patient with mild cardiovascular disease (e.g., a patient with mild to moderate hypertension):

1. precordial or esophageal stethoscopy
2. oscilloscopic electrocardiography (V_5 lead recommended)
3. sphygmomanometry, using detection of Korotkoff's sounds or a Doppler ultrasonic signal
4. temperature probe

Patient with moderate cardiovascular disease (e.g., severe hypertension, arteriosclerotic vascular disease, coronary artery disease, valvular heart disease, or the patient with mild cardiovascular disease who is undergoing major intra-abdominal or intrathoracic surgery):

1. precordial or esophageal stethoscopy
2. oscilloscopic electrocardiography with V_5 and lead II, if possible
3. direct measurement of intra-arterial pressure, using an indwelling arterial cannula and transducer-oscilloscopic display
4. central venous pressure, water manometer acceptable
5. temperature, either esophageal or rectal
6. urinary output, especially if large fluid and volume shifts are anticipated

Patient with severe cardiovascular disease and cardiac surgery patients:

1. esophageal stethoscopy
2. oscilloscopic electrocardiography with simultaneous V_5 and lead II
3. intra-arterial pressure measurement, using indwelling arterial catheter and transducer-oscilloscopic display
4. central venous pressure with transducer and oscilloscopic display
5. pulmonary artery pressure and pulmonary capillary wedge pressure, using a pulmonary artery catheter
6. cardiac output, using the thermodilution technique via the pulmonary artery catheter
7. esophageal, rectal, or nasopharyngeal temperature
8. urinary output via indwelling catheter
9. continuous on-line measurement of intra-arterial oxygen and carbon dioxide tensions, if equipment available

SUMMARY

Cardiovascular data can provide the anesthesiologist with very valuable information that enables him to take better care of his patient. This information will prove even more valuable if the following few rules are followed: (1) do not be mesmerized, confused, or preoccupied by complex equipment, (2) do not avoid paying direct attention to your patient, (3) remember to use what will provide clinically useful information and heed this information, and (4) remember that electronic monitoring is not *always* superior to other methods.

BIBLIOGRAPHY

Bedford, R. F.: *Percutaneous radial-artery cannulation—increased safety using Teflon catheters.* Anesthesiology 42:219, 1975.

Bedford, R. F.: *Long-term radial-artery cannulation: effects on subsequent vessel function.* Crit. Care Med. 6:64, 1978.

Bedford, R. F.: *Radial-arterial function following percutaneous cannulation with 18- and 20-gauge catheters.* Anesthesiology 47:37, 1978.

Bedford, R. F.: *Wrist circumference predicts the risk of radial-arterial occlusion after cannulation.* Anesthesiology 48:377, 1978.

Bedford, R. F., and Wollman, H.: *Complications of percutaneous radial-artery cannulation: an objective prospective study in man.* Anesthesiology 38:228, 1973.

Brodsky, J. B.: *A simple method to determine potency of the ulnar artery intraoperatively prior to radial-artery cannulation.* Anesthesiology 42:626, 1975.

Buchbinder, N., and Ganz, W.: *Hemodynamic monitoring: invasive techniques.* Anesthesiology 45:146, 1976.

Defalque, R. J.: *The subclavian route: a critical review of the world literature up to 1970.* Der Anaesthetist 21:325, 1972.

Defalque, R. J.: *Percutaneous catheterization of the internal jugular vein.* Anesth. Analg. (Cleve.) 53:116, 1974.

Downs, J. B., Chapman, and Hawkins, I. F.: *Prolonged radial-artery catheterization: an evaluation of heparinized catheters and continuous irrigation.* Arch. Surg. 108:671, 1974.

Downs, J. B., Rackstein, A. D., Klein, E. F., et al.: *Hazards of radial-artery catheterization.* Anesthesiology 38:283, 1973.

Gardner, R. M., Schwartz, R., Wong, H. E., et al.: *Percutaneous indwelling radial-artery catheters for monitoring cardiovascular function: prospective study of the risk of thrombosis and infection.* N. Engl. J. Med. 390:1227, 1974.

Greenhow, D. E.: *Incorrect performance of Allen's test—ulnar artery flow erroneously presumed inadequate.* Anesthesiology 37:356, 357, 1972.

Hartong, J., and Dixon, R. S.: *Monitoring resuscitation of the injured patient.* J.A.M.A. 237:242, 1977.

Johnstone, R. E., and Greenhow, D. E.: *Catheterization of the dorsalis pedis artery.* Anesthesiology 39: 654, 1973.

Kaplan, J. A., Dunbar, R. W., and Hatcher, C. R.: *Diagnostic value with a V_5 precordial electrographic lead: a case report.* Anesth. Analg. (Cleve.) 57:364, 1978.

Kim, J. M., Arakawa, K., and Bliss, J.: *Arterial cannulation: factors in the development of occlusion.* Anesth. Analg. (Cleve.) 54:836, 1975.

Lappas, D.G., Lell, W. A., Gabel, J. C., et al.: *Indirect measurement of left-atrial pressure in surgical patients—pulmonary-capillary wedge and pulmonary-artery diastolic pressures compared with left-atrial pressure.* Anesthesiology 38:394, 1973.

Lappas, D. G., Powell, W. M. J., and Daggett, W. M.: *Cardiac dysfunction in the perioperative period: pathophysiology, diagnosis and treatment.* Anesthesiology 47:117, 1977.

Pace, N. L.: *A critique of flow-directed pulmonary arterial catheterization.* Anesthesiology 47:455, 1977.

Price, S. R., Sullivan, R. L., and Hackel, A.: *Percutaneous catheterization of the internal jugular vein in infants and children.* Anesthesiology 44:170, 1976.

Prys-Roberts, C.: *Monitoring of the cardiovascular system.* In Saidman, L. J., and Smith, N. T. (eds.): *Monitoring in Anesthesia.* John Wiley & Sons, Inc., New York, 1978.

Ramanathan, S., Chalon, J., and Turndorf, H.: *Determining patency of palmar arches by retrograde radial pulsation.* Anesthesiology 42:756, 1975.

Reitan, J. A.: *Noninvasive monitoring.* In Saidman, L. J., and Smith, N. T. (eds.): *Monitoring in Anesthesia.* John Wiley & Sons, Inc., 1978, pp. 85–125.

Samii, K., Conseiller, C., and Viars, P.: *Central venous pressure and pulmonary wedge pressure: a comparative study in anesthetized surgical patients.* Arch. Surg. 111:1122, 1976.

Swan, H. J. C., Ganz, W., Forrester, J., et al.: *Catheterization of the heart in man with use of a flow-directed balloon-tipped catheter.* N. Engl. J. Med. 283:447, 1970.

Weber, D. R., and Arens, J.: *Use of cephalic and basilic veins for introduction of central venous catheters.* Anesthesiology 38:389, 1973.

ANESTHESIA AND CONGENITAL HEART DEFECTS

Hugh D. Allen, M.D.

Anesthesiologists at large centers are frequently consulted to administer anesthesia for noncardiac surgery in a premature or newborn infant with a congenital heart anomaly. Since many of these anesthetics must be performed by noncardiac anesthetists, knowledge of the pathophysiology of these conditions is a prerequisite for rational management of anesthesia. Dr. Hugh Allen has a great depth of experience in diagnosis and treatment of this constellation of syndromes. His outline, although not intended to be comprehensive, details the cardinal problems relevant to anesthesia in several congenital cardiac problems. The interested clinician is referred to standard texts for more complete descriptions. Needless to say, management of these infants is challenging and tests the mettle of the anesthesiologist.

Burnell R. Brown, Jr.

Congenital heart disease occurs in 6 to 7 of 1000 live births. Defects can range in severity from barely detectable to incompatible with survival. The anesthesiologist not dealing with closed or open heart procedures may encounter children with milder forms (or treated forms) of congenital heart disease on a fairly regular basis if he has a significant pediatric component in his practice. Accordingly, this chapter is directed to the practicing anesthesiologist who will be treating children with congenital heart disease for needs unrelated to their cardiac lesion. It will include a general discussion of the types of congenital heart lesions that the anesthesiologist will most likely encounter and will also discuss general principles of anesthetic management related to specific anomalies, with emphasis and caveats, where applicable.

Congenital heart disease is classified in many ways. One of the most useful classifications for the clinician is based upon the presence or absence of cyanosis. Acyanotic congenital heart disease is more common.

ACYANOTIC CONGENITAL HEART DISEASE

Two major subclassifications of acyanotic heart disease exist: left-to-right shunt lesions and valve lesions. With certain unusual anatomic and physiologic circumstances, patients with acyanotic diseases can become cyanotic, but only one of these variations will be addressed.

Left-to-Right Shunts

The three most common left-to-right shunt lesions are ventricular septal defect, atrial septal defect, and patent ductus arteriosus.

VENTRICULAR SEPTAL DEFECT

Ventricular septal defects (VSD) occur in about 20 percent of children with congenital heart disease and are the most common congenital heart defect. Clinical expression can be quite variable, ranging from inconsequential to severe congestive heart failure. This gamut of presentations is due to the size of the defect itself and the relationship between the resistances met by the left and right ventricles. If a patient has a large ventricular septal defect, associated with coarctation of the aorta (high left ventricular afterload resistance) and low pulmonary resistance, left-to-right shunting will be massive, and increased pulmonary blood flow will, upon re-entering the heart, cause considerable dilation of the overloaded left ventricle. Obviously, this is the common denominator of heart failure. On the other hand, if there is high right ventricular afterload resistance (e.g., pulmonary stenosis, a surgically placed pulmonary artery band, or pulmonary vascular obstructive disease—PVOD) and normal systemic resistance, very little left-to-right shunting occurs. If right ventricular afterload resistance exceeds that presented to the left ventricle, blood will flow from the right ventricle to the left ventricle through the VSD (a right-to-left shunt). This blood, mixed with the oxygenated left ventricular blood, is then ejected into the aorta. Aortic PO_2 is lower than normal and, if low enough, produces visible cyanosis. A VSD with high pulmonary arterial resistance (PVOD) and a resultant right-to-left shunt is called the Eisenmenger complex.

Most patients with a VSD, however, have a small defect with little left-to-right shunting. Few VSDs require surgical closure and, of the remainder, 80 percent will close spontaneously at some time. The patient with a moderate to small VSD is the one most often encountered in anesthetic practice. If the child shows no signs or symptoms of congestive heart failure (and is not taking digitalis), the anesthetic risk should be no more than that for the average pediatric patient, except for an increased chance of postoperative bacterial endocarditis.

In contrast, the patient with Eisenmenger complex represents a grave anesthetic risk. The pulmonary resistance is high and generally nonreactive, and it possesses a right-to-left intraventricular shunt. This patient is inoperable from a corrective standpoint. A decrease in systemic resistance, or an increase in pulmonary resistance, will accentuate the shunt and decrease the pulmonary blood flow. If these patients become hypoxic, they develop acidosis, which is very difficult to reverse. Arrhythmias are much more likely to occur in the presence of acidosis, hypoxia, and hypercarbia, especially if the patient is taking digitalis preparations.

The anesthesiologist must be very cautious with a patient with Eisenmenger complex. Is the surgical procedure really necessary? Does the patient have a history of arrhythmias? Is he taking cardiac glycosides? Was there pulmonary vascular reactivity at his last catheterization? (This is unlikely since that type of patient usually is a suitable candidate for cardiac repair.) As mentioned, all steps should be taken to avoid hypoxia during induction and anesthesia, and after surgery. Withholding the last few digoxin doses is probably prudent from a standpoint of reducing serious risks of arrhythmia, but this must be weighed against the need for a positive inotropic drug. Preoperative hydration should be carefully maintained. Because these patients have right-to-left intracardiac shunts, avoid flushing clots or air from the intravenous line. Paradoxical embolism can occur. Induction and tracheal intubation must be smooth in order to prevent increases in myocardial demand. Avoid systemic hypotension and, if anything, allow the patient to be somewhat systemically hypertensive during the procedure. Halothane lowers peripheral resistance, whereas ketamine usually does not; thus, ketamine in conjunction with a neuromuscular blocker and nitrous oxide may be preferable. Precautions against endocarditis must be employed. Last, always reconsider the question, ''Is the surgical procedure really necessary?''

ATRIAL SEPTAL DEFECT

Atrial septal defects (ASD) are an extremely common congenital cardiac abnormality. Most common is the secundum type, although defects can also occur at the foramen ovale area, at the superior vena cava-atrial junction (sinus venosus type), or at the central fibrous body of the heart derived from the endocardial cushion. The last-named are the ostium primum defects and are usually associated with cleft mitral valves.

Children with uncomplicated ASDs are usually asymptomatic. Although pulmonary blood flow is increased and right ventricular volume overload exists, the pediatric patient seldom has pulmonary hypertension or congestive heart failure. As the disease progresses into the patient's adulthood, pulmonary arterial pressure becomes elevated and the heart may fail, but this is uncommon, since most of those defects are repaired before the child enters school.

Those patients with cleft mitral valves (associated with the primum ASD) may have mitral insufficiency as a jet lesion. The risk of endocarditis is accordingly higher in these patients than in those with secundum ASDs. Valvular pulmonary stenosis occasionally accompanies the secundum ASD, and these patients (with a pulmonary jet lesion) will also require endocarditic prophylaxis for surgery. If the question of endocarditis coverage is in doubt, it is probably prudent to treat.

Anesthetic risk for the patient with an atrial septal defect is probably no higher than that for the normal population. No specific anesthetic drugs can be recommended or contraindicated.

PATENT DUCTUS ARTERIOSUS

Patent ductus arteriosus (PDA) is a more common problem in neonatal pediatrics, since premature infants are now surviving the associated respiratory distress syndrome (RDS) because of marked improvements in neonatal care. Patent ductus arteriosus frequently accompanies the RDS problem and may complicate it considerably. Large patent ductus arterioses will have been either medically or surgically treated by the time these patients are seen for elective surgery, but smaller patent ductus arterioses will still be present. Premature infants who "graduate" from the nursery often have strabismus or hernias and may require surgery; this is the population with which the anesthesiologist will most likely deal. The likelihood of anesthetizing an older child with a PDA is remote, since most patients are corrected by the time they are one year old.

Anesthetic risk for the patient with a small PDA is probably no higher than that for the general population, but endocarditis prophylaxis is recommended.

GENERAL COMMENT

If the patient has a fairly large left-to-right shunt (VSD, PDA, or ASD), with some pulmonary edema, continuous positive end expiratory pressure will help to avoid intraoperative and postoperative ventilation/perfusion inequalities. Avoid high ambient oxygen levels, since pulmonary resistance will be decreased and pulmonary flow will increase accordingly, complicating an already high flow situation. Similarly, avoid anesthetic drugs that increase pulmonary blood flow or systemic resistance (Table 1). The patient with a large left-to-right shunt generally requires intensive postoperative pulmonary management. Do not be in too much of a hurry to extubate this patient's trachea.

Table 1. Effects of Agents.

Increase Pulmonary Resistance
  Hypoxia
  Promethazine
  Cyclopropane
  Diethyl ether
  Hypercarbia
Decrease Pulmonary Resistance
  Oxygen
  Tolazoline
Increase Systemic Resistance
  Phenylephrine
  Methoxamine
  Ephedrine
  Cyclopropane
  Ketamine
Decrease Systemic Resistance
  Halothane
  Thiopental
  Spinal anesthesia
  Tolazoline
  Isoproterenol
  Nitroprusside
Increase Myocardial Contractility
  Digitalis glycosides
  Isoproterenol
  Dopamine
Cause Myocardial Depression
  Propranolol
  Cyclopropane
  Ketamine (because of tachycardia)
  Halogenated inhalation anesthetics

Valvular Heart Disease

Most patients with valvular heart disease are not cyanotic. Valvular disease is a matter of either stenosis, insufficiency, or both. Since mitral stenosis and tricuspid stenosis are extremely rare lesions in the pediatric patient, they will not be discussed. The most common stenotic lesions involve the aortic and pulmonary valves.

AORTIC STENOSIS

The aortic valve is normally tricuspid. Owing to embryologic failure of the raphae to separate, unicuspid or bicuspid valves can develop. These are often stenotic, but the bicuspid valves can be nonstenotic depending upon the degree of commissural fusion. The usual gross appearance of a congenitally deformed and stenotic valve resembles that of a windsock. The opening dictates the amount of left ventricular pressure necessary to deliver an appropriate stroke volume and cardiac output over a given amount of ejection time. If the narrowing is severe, significant afterload is created, and the ventricle will undergo hypertrophy.

Coronary blood flow occurs in diastole. The amount of flow per gram of cardiac tissue depends upon the patency of the coronary arteries, the thickness of the muscle to be perfused, and the pressure gradient between the aortic diastolic pressure and the left ventricular diastolic pressure.

In mild aortic stenosis, no problem of any degree will be encountered. However, if the valve is severely stenotic, less blood may be ejected and muscle (because of hypertrophy) may not be perfused. This is especially notable during stress, when peripheral oxygen demands are increased but the stroke output is fixed, owing to limitations imposed by the stenosis. Cardiac output is thus decreased absolutely and relatively. As cardiac tissue demands oxygen and stroke output is relatively decreased, the thickened myocardium is underperfused, especially at the subendocardial area. Some cardiac failure can occur, which results in elevation of ventricular diastolic pressure. This causes a decrease in the gradient between aortic and left ventricular diastolic pressures, and coronary flow is decreased, leading to more subendocardial ischemia. This vicious cycle can lead to severe underperfusion or to cardiac irritability and arrhythmias. Fainting can occur in the awake state, owing to cerebral hypoxia or to arrhythmias. Aortic valve stenosis of a greater than minor degree should be corrected before any elective noncardiac surgical procedures are performed.

Prior to surgery the patient should be fully prepared emotionally and sedated to help relieve anxiety. Induction and endotracheal intubation should obviously be smooth. Thiopental may be a good choice of induction in the older child. Doses of drugs that markedly alter afterload (in either direction) should be avoided. Morphine and the nitrous oxide-oxygen-muscle relaxant sequence might be good anesthetic choices. Higher oxygen levels than ambient are preferable. Careful monitoring of electrocardiographic leads II, III, AVF, or V_6 for ST–T changes or arrhythmias is mandatory, if not precluded by thoracic surgery. Intraoperative and postoperative hypoxia and acidosis must be avoided. Appropriate antibiotic prophylaxis against endocarditis should be given.

AORTIC INSUFFICIENCY

Aortic valve insufficiency results in diastolic regurgitation of aortic blood back into the left ventricle. The left ventricle is thus overloaded. The extent of the overload in volume is determined by the aortic diastolic pressure, the degree of valve deformity, wall tension (or compliance) of the left ventricle, and left ventricular diastolic pressure. Coronary flow may be affected by the left ventricular diastolic pressure and the extent of left ventricular muscle mass (hypertrophy).

During anesthesia, the patient with mild aortic insufficiency will probably present no problem. However, the patient with severe insufficiency, a markedly dilated left ventricle, and subendocardial ischemia may be prone to arrhythmias and/or worsening failure during general anesthesia. Anesthetic adjuvants that increase systemic afterload should be avoided. In fact, reduction of afterload may be beneficial. Intraoperative and postoperative electrocardiographic monitoring is necessary. Precautions against endocarditis should be employed.

PULMONARY VALVE STENOSIS

Untreated valvular pulmonary stenosis is seldom severe enough to present much problem to the anesthesiologist. If it is severe, however, pulmonary blood flow may be limited during periods of stress. Thus, myocardial depressants should be avoided and tracheal intubation for induction should be smooth. Antibiotic prophylaxis for endocarditis should be given.

PULMONARY VALVULAR INSUFFICIENCY

Mild pulmonary valvular insufficiency results in some right ventricular volume overload, but generally presents no problem to the anesthesiologist. A more severe form, the absent pulmonary valve (usually associated with a ventricular septal defect), is ac-

Table 2. Dosages for Antibiotic Prophylaxis Against Endocarditis.

FOR DENTAL PROCEDURES AND SURGERY OF THE UPPER
RESPIRATORY TRACT
Regimen A—Penicillin
1. Parenteral–oral combined
   Children: Aqueous crystalline penicillin G (30,000 units/kg
   intramuscularly), *mixed with* procaine penicillin G (600,000 units
   intramuscularly). Timing of doses for children is the same as for
   adults. For children less than 60 lb, the dose of penicillin V is 250
   mg orally every 6 hours for 8 doses.
2. Oral
   Children: Penicillin V (2.0 g orally 30 minutes to 1 hour prior to
   procedure and then 500 mg orally every 6 hours for 8 doses). For
   children less than 60 lb, use 1.0 g orally 30 minutes to 1 hour prior
   to the procedure and then 250 mg orally every 6 hours for 8
   doses.
For Patients Allergic to Penicillin
   Use either vancomycin (see Regimen B)
                            or
   Children: Erythromycin (20 mg/kg orally 1½ to 2 hours prior to
   the procedure and then 10 mg/kg every 6 hours for 8 doses).
Regimen B—Penicillin Plus Streptomycin
   Children: Aqueous crystalline penicillin G (30,000 units/kg
   intramuscularly), *mixed with* Procaine penicillin G (600,000 units
   intramuscularly) *plus* Streptomycin (20 mg/kg intramuscularly).
   Timing of doses for children is the same as for adults. For
   children less than 60 lb, the recommended oral dose of penicillin
   V is 250 mg every 6 hours for 8 doses.
For Patients Allergic to Penicillin
   Children: Vancomycin (20 mg/kg given intravenously over 30
   minutes to 1 hour) *plus* Streptomycin (20 mg/kg intramuscularly).
   Timing of doses for children is the same as for adults.
FOR GASTROINTESTINAL AND GENITOURINARY TRACT SURGERY
AND INSTRUMENTATION
   Children: Aqueous crystalline penicillin G (30,000 units/kg
   intramuscularly or intravenously)
                            or
   Ampicillin (50 mg/kg intramuscularly or intravenously)
                           plus
   Gentamicin (2.0 mg/kg intramuscularly or intravenously)
                            or
   Streptomycin (20 mg/kg intramuscularly). Timing of doses for
   children is the same as for adults.
For Patients Allergic to Penicillin
   Children: Vancomycin (20 mg/kg given intravenously over 30
   minutes to 1 hour) *plus* Streptomycin (20 mg/kg intramuscularly).
   Timing of doses for children is the same as for adults.

companied by very dilated branch pulmonary arteries. These can impinge upon bronchi, constricting them in a hemodynamic vise and making pulmonary toilet very difficult. These patients have frequent bouts of pneumonitis and may have impaired pulmonary function.

Pulmonary function testing and careful examination to rule out pneumonia are important preoperative requirements in adequately evaluating these patients. Avoid intraoperative dessication of bronchial secretions; careful postoperative pulmonary care is mandatory. Again, care should be exercised when negative inotropic drugs are required (Table 2). Antibiotic prophylaxis against endocarditis should be given.

CYANOTIC CONGENITAL HEART DISEASE

Cyanotic congenital heart disease is subclassified upon the basis of roentgenographic evidence of decreased or increased pulmonary blood flow. Clinically visible cyanosis results from greater or lesser addition of systemic venous (desaturated) blood to greater or lesser amounts of pulmonary venous (oxygenated) blood. Mixing can occur at any level, for example, precardiac (anomalous pulmonary venous drainage), atrial, ventricular, or great vessel. Such mixing constitutes the well-known right-to-left shunt.

CYANOTIC LESIONS WITH DECREASED PULMONARY BLOOD FLOW

Tetralogy of Fallot

The commonest cyanotic heart lesion is tetralogy of Fallot. Classically, tetralogy of Fallot is a conotruncal abnormality wherein the aorta straddles (overrides) the interventricular septum, there is a ventricular septal defect just below the overriding aorta, and the right ventricular outflow tract is obstructed to a greater or lesser extent at the pulmonary valvular or right ventricular infundibular level (or both). Narrowing of the right ventricular outflow tract leads to a resistance higher than that of the systemic circuit; some returning systemic venous blood will shunt from the right ventricle via the VSD to the systemic circulation. It will then mix with oxygenated blood and result in cyanosis. Further, as some of the returned systemic venous blood is shunted right to left before the remainder enters the pulmonary artery, pulmonary blood flow is decreased.

In addition to this classical form of tetralogy of Fallot, patients may have somewhat different anatomic defects with generally similar flow characteristics. For example, a patient can have pulmonary valve atresia or severe pulmonary stenosis, a ventricular septal defect in the membranous portion of the septum, no aortic override, and right ventricular hypertrophy secondary to the right ventricular pressure overload. This will bring about no (or decreased) pulmonary blood flow and right-to-left shunting at the ventricular level. Thus, identical "tetralogy physiology" is possible with different anatomic presentations.

The clinical status of a patient with tetralogy of Fallot is largely dictated by the amount of pulmonary blood flow. Too little pulmonary flow results in insufficient delivery of oxygen to tissues (hypoxia), anaerobic metabolism, acidosis, and death. Since pulmonary flow is dependent upon a balance between systemic and pulmonary resistance, alterations in these resistances can lead to symptomatology. For example, exercise, a meal, a warm bath, arising from sleep, or certain anesthetic agents can decrease systemic resistance. If pulmonary outflow resistance is fixed, systemic flow will increase, the right-to-left shunt will increase, and pulmonary blood flow will accordingly decrease. The ambulatory child with tetralogy will respond to this situation by squatting, which increases systemic resistance, decreases the right-to-left shunt, and increases pulmonary blood flow. If this does not occur, the patient will evidence increasing cyanosis and may faint. This is called a tetrad spell. If pulmonary flow is not increased by some mechanism, acidosis and death can result.

Another mechanism producing decreased pulmonary blood flow in tetralogy is an increase in the resistance of the right ventricle. Fixed valvular pulmonary stenosis will offer little dynamic change in resistance, but subvalvular (infundibular) resistance can. Infundibular spasm can occur with manipulation of catheters during cardiac catheterization, with administration of cardiotonic drugs (digoxin), and at unpredictable times. An increase in pulmonary arteriolar tone can also increase right ventricular afterload. This is most commonly seen during episodes of hypoxia or when the child is acutely exposed to increased altitude (driving up a mountain or flying in poorly pressurized aircraft). Again, the balance of resistances is shifted, right-to-left flow is increased, and pulmonary flow is decreased.

Treatment of these spells is directed toward increasing systemic resistance and decreasing right ventricular afterload, thus increasing pulmonary blood flow. If the patient is too young or too faint to squat, force his knees into his abdomen and press, which causes some aortic and iliac compression and increased systemic resistance. Since peripheral perfusion is decreased, drugs should be administered intravenously. As many drugs are less active in an acidotic environment, intravenous alkalinization with sodium bicarbonate may be necessary. Drugs that increase peripheral resistance (e.g., methoxamine, phenylephrine, ephedrine) may be useful. Plasma expanders should be used. Propranolol can be given intravenously in order to produce myocardial depression (and therefore relax infundibular spasm). Remember that the intravenous dose of propranolol (0.1 mg/kg I.V.) is one tenth the oral dose. Although its mechanism is uncertain, intravenous morphine (0.14 to 0.10 mg/kg) is very useful for therapy of tetrad spells. Administration of oxygen by mask may decrease pulmonary vascular resistance, but it has little other usefulness. A small amount of pulmonary flow will be better oxygenated, but this is frequently inconsequential. Too many minutes of treatment of cyanotic episodes have been lost while the effects of oxygen by mask were awaited and no other therapy was employed. Finally, if no response has taken place in spite of the described therapy, emergency surgical shunting of the systemic artery to the pulmonary artery or definitive surgical repair may be necessary for survival.

Patients with reactive infundibula are more prone to have tetrad spells, particularly if they are infants and small children. In contrast, surviving tetralogy patients with complete pulmonary valve atresia will have already had shunt surgery or complete repair. Since their pulmonary circulation is completely dependent on a patent ductus arteriosus, if the ductus closes, they will not survive. Most are recognized in the nursery and undergo emergency catheterization and surgery immediately. The other group, those with pulmonary stenosis and infundibular stenosis, may be acyanotic at birth, but worsen with time as the infundibulum progressively narrows. They evidence increasing cyanosis and develop rising hemoglobin levels. Those who are relatively iron-deficient (higher than normal hemoglobin level, but abnormal red blood cell indices, with decreased mean corpuscular hemoglobin levels) are most prone to tetrad spells.

The anesthesiologist may well be faced with such a patient, who will undergo noncardiac surgery. Several precautions should be taken. First, procedures should be done in a center where a pediatric cardiologist, cardiovascular surgeon, and cardiac support facilities are available. The patient should be premedicated with atropine and morphine, which may help abort a tetrad spell. Hypoxia must be avoided during induction of anesthesia. Endotracheal intubation must be atraumatic. Avoid anesthetic agents that decrease systemic resistance (e.g., deep halothane, thiopental, caudal) and avoid agents (e.g., ether) that increase pulmonary resistance. Pulmonary vascular resistance is not the major resistance component, but may play a minor role in tetralogy. Avoid positive inotropic drugs that can cause infundibular spasm (e.g., isoproterenol, digoxin). An acceptable regimen is N_2O-O_2/light halothane, muscle relaxant, and 0.1 mg/kg morphine. A heavy-dose narcotic anesthetic is quite good. Other necessary precautions include avoiding flushing air or clots from the intravenous lines, as these patients shunt right to left and may paradoxically embolize these materials. The patient with a high hemoglobin level should not be dehydrated, since red blood cell sludging may occur. These patients may have a clotting disorder. Prothrombin time, partial thromboplastin time, and platelet count should be determined preoperatively. Phlebotomy is sometimes necessary to help correct these abnormalities. If the patient has relative iron deficiency anemia, and if the procedure is elective, the procedure should be deferred and iron therapy given until the patient is no longer relatively anemic. Precautions against endocarditis should be rigorously applied. Last, anesthesia should be given to this type of patient only by an experienced anesthesiologist. This includes the endotracheal intubation procedure, intraoperative management, and postoperative care. Obviously, in these patients, the benefit of the procedure must be weighed in comparison with risk. A preoperative consultation between the child's cardiologist, surgeon, and anesthesiologist would probably be useful.

Anesthesia in the patient who has had a shunt procedure, or in the patient who has had a complete repair, is obviously much less complicated. Here, anesthetic precautions are less stringent, but precautions against endocarditis should still be employed. Further, in the patient with a surgical shunt, intracardiac right-to-left shunting still exists, and caution against paradoxical embolization should be rigorously applied.

Pulmonary Atresia with Intact Ventricular Septum, Hypoplastic Right Ventricle, and Tricuspid Atresia

All these lesions share a common physiology. Pulmonary blood flow is generally reduced. The right ventricle is bypassed by the returning systemic venous blood, which shunts from the right atrium to the left atrium via a patent foramen ovale or an atrial septal defect. This blood mixes with the left atrial blood (the returned pulmonary flow) and enters the left ventricle and aorta. If the patient has tricuspid atresia, a ventricular septal defect is usually present and some of the left ventricular blood is shunted into the pulmonary circuit. Otherwise, pulmonary flow is totally dependent upon blood shunted from the aorta to the pulmonary artery. In the newborn this is accomplished by a patent ductus arteriosus. By the time the anesthesiologist sees this patient for a noncardiac surgical procedure, a surgical shunting of the systemic artery to the pulmonary artery almost necessarily will have been performed.

The general anesthetic precautions that applied to the tetralogy patient who had a surgical shunt apply here. As there is an intracardiac right-to-left shunt, paradoxical embolization must be avoided. Precautions against endocarditis must be rigorously applied. If questions exist, preoperative consultation with a pediatric cardiologist is probably in order.

CYANOTIC LESIONS WITH INCREASED PULMONARY BLOOD FLOW

These lesions are often called admixture lesions because a common preaortic mix of systemic venous and pulmonary venous blood takes place. Defects include total anomalous pulmonary venous drainage, single atrium, single ventricle (without pulmonary stenosis), double outlet right ventricle, transposition of the great arteries, and truncus arteriosus. Principles of anesthetic management in all these disorders are similar and will be discussed at the end of this section.

Total Anomalous Pulmonary Venous Drainage

Embryologic diversion of the returning pulmonary blood flow away from the left atrium results in eventual pulmonary venous drainage into the right atrium. This can be accomplished via many routes—by the coronary sinus, by a vertical vein to the innominate vein, directly into the right atrium, or subdiaphragmatically to the portal system. The pulmonary venous blood mixes with the returning systemic venous blood. This mixed blood is then recirculated to the lungs, with the systemic cardiac output passing into the left atrium via an atrial septal defect. The degree of peripheral cyanosis is dictated by the amount of pulmonary blood flow that mixes with the systemic blood. Factors then affecting cyanosis include pulmonary vascular resistance, obstruction to pulmonary venous return, size of the atrial septal defect, and left ventricular compliance.

Single Atrium, Single Ventricle, and Double Outlet Right Ventricle

Each of these lesions allows mixing at a different cardiac level. Patients with single atrium are seldom cyanotic, unless some obstruction to right ventricular inflow exists. The same is true for patients with single ventricle, where streaming takes place. The patient is usually acyanotic unless obstruction to right ventricular outflow or alteration in great vessel location exists, as in double outlet right ventricle, in which both great vessels arise from the right ventricle. Cyanosis is especially apparent in the latter condition, when the pulmonary artery rather than the aorta is related to the ventricular septal defect and thus receives the shunted left ventricular streaming, and the aorta receives deoxygenated systemic venous blood.

Transposition of the Great Vessels

Transposition of the great vessels is a condition in which the aorta arises from the right ventricle and the pulmonary artery arises from the left ventricle. (Ventricular inversion will not be included in this discussion.) The complex can be accompanied by a ventricular septal defect, with or without subpulmonic narrowing, but often is associated with an intact ventricular septum. Since circulation in this situation is parallel (systemic vein → right atrium → right ventricle → aorta systemic vein and pulmonary vein → left atrium → left ventricle → pulmonary artery → pulmonary vein), mixing must occur at some site in order to assure survival. This lesion is usually diagnosed in infancy (usually in the first several hours of life). A balloon atrial septostomy (Rashkind procedure) is then performed. A catheter is placed into the left atrium via a patent foramen ovale. A balloon on the tip of the catheter is then inflated and forcefully jerked into the right atrium, tearing the interatrial septum. Mixing of pulmonary venous and systemic venous blood can then take place via this created atrial septal defect. Operative rerouting of the atrial circulation (Mustard procedure or Senning procedure) is then accomplished some time between the newborn period and 1 to 2 years of age.

Truncus Arteriosus

Truncus arteriosus is a conotruncal defect anatomically similar to tetralogy except that the pulmonary artery arises at truncal (great vessel) level instead of from the heart. The pulmonary artery origin is valveless and generally nonstenotic, and thus pulmonary flow is nonrestricted. A ventricular septal defect (in the conotruncal septal area) is invariably present. Mixing of systemic and pulmonary venous flow occurs at high ventricular and truncal levels.

General Comment

General anesthetic considerations in these lesions center around meticulous care to avoid paradoxical embolization of air or particulate materials from intravenous lines through the areas of right-to-left shunting into the systemic circulation. Further, doses of drugs that alter pulmonary or systemic resistances to any great degree should be avoided, as the circulation may be fairly delicately balanced. Many of these patients are taking cardiac glycosides, and careful attempts to monitor and avoid arrhythmias should be employed. Antibiotic prophylaxis against endocarditis should be given.

CONCLUSION

In order to provide ideal care for the pediatric patient with heart disease who is at risk for surgery and anesthesia, the procedure should be performed at a center that is adequately staffed. Personnel and facilities should include a pediatric cardiologist, a cardiovascular surgeon, a pediatric surgeon, an anesthesiologist who is well versed in cardiovascular and pediatric problems, a pediatric pulmonologist, a respiratory therapy group, and an adequately staffed pediatric intensive care unit. All back-up laboratory facilities, including microchemistry laboratory, hematology laboratory, blood bank, cardiac catheterization laboratory, cardiovascular operating room and staff, electrocardiography, and x-ray and echocardiographic laboratories, should be available on a 24-hour basis. If you have doubt, obtain a preoperative consultation with the pediatric cardiologist. Obviously, this is not necessary in the patient with a small ventricular septal defect or trivial pulmonary stenosis, or in the patient who may already have had a preoperative visit to a pediatric cardiology clinic.

If the patient has a left-to-right shunt, avoid doses of drugs that increase pulmonary blood flow by decreasing pulmonary resistance. If the patient has a right-to-left shunt, determine why. Never get behind in oxygenation of the patient with the Eisenmenger complex and avoid acidosis in these patients. Do not allow systemic hypotension. In patients with tetralogy, prevent infundibular spasm and be prepared to treat a tetrad spell. (See text for a detailed discussion of caveats.) Avoid paradoxic embolization. If the patient has significant left ventricular outflow obstruction, myocardial (coronary) blood flow is already compromised. Eschew doses of drugs that cause further myocardial depression.

Arrhythmias may occur and are usually in the form of bradycardias. Atropine administered intravenously is very useful here (even if the patient was premedicated with atropine). Specific arrhythmias otherwise require specific therapy.

The newborn presents a particularly challenging anesthetic problem. In addition to routine monitoring during anesthesia, careful attention to temperature control is necessary. Infants have a nonshivering thermogenesis that is chemical and results in a lactic acidosis. An imbalance between the sympathetic and parasympathetic systems exists, and smaller infants are more "vagal" than adults. Thus, stress is shown as a bradycardia (especially in premature infants). Careful attention should be given to color (and color of blood in the operating field), blood loss (including lab specimens—an infant has 80 ml of circulating blood volume per kg body weight), clotting, heart rate, change in murmur, arterial pressure, central venous pressure, PO_2, arterial blood gases, ECG, electrolytes, calcium and glucose levels, and specific examinations as otherwise indicated.

Antibiotic prophylaxis against bacterial endocarditis must be employed in nearly every lesion. This especially applies to contaminated surgery. Table 2 provides specific doses and procedures.

Finally, the psychological status of your patient should be considered. Children fantasize. Some of the pediatric heart patients' worst fantasies have already been realized in the cardiac catheterization laboratory or in the operating room or the intensive care unit. Be attuned to the patients' and parents' concerns and act accordingly. We find play room therapy quite useful. The patient explains to a nurse or therapist what is going to happen to him by demonstration on a doll. This can be quite revealing. Be honest with children, but don't be brusque or cruel. They are a great group of people. Excellent care is their right and your privilege to give.

BIBLIOGRAPHY

Hanson, D. D.: *Anesthesia.* In Sade, R. M., Cosgrove, D. M., and Castaneda, A. R. (eds.): *Infant and Child Care in Heart Surgery.* Chicago, Year Book Medical Publishers, Inc., 1977

Kaplan, E. L.: *Prevention of bacterial endocarditis.* Circulation 56:139A, 1977, tables on pp. 140A, 141A, and 142A.

Moss, A. J., Adams, F. H., and Emmanouilides, G. C. (eds.): *Heart Disease in Infants, Children and Adolescents,* ed. 6. Baltimore, Williams & Wilkins Co., 1978.

Rudolph, A. M.: *Congenital Diseases of the Heart.* Chicago, Year Book Medical Publishers, Inc., 1974.

Wunderlich, J. B.: *Anesthetic management.* In Billing, D. M., and Kreidberg, M. B. (eds.): *The Management of Neonates and Infants with Congenital Heart Disease.* New York, Grune & Stratton, 1973.

POSTOPERATIVE PROGNOSIS IN PATIENTS WITH PRE-EXISTING HEART DISEASE

Richard B. Knapp, M.D.

Dr. Knapp has written a chapter dedicated to a relevant discussion of risk factors involved in anesthesia and surgery for the patient with coronary insufficiency, with and without previous myocardial infarction. Obviously, it is impossible to inform precisely any particular patient of his or her possibility of reinfarction or death. However, there now exists a substantial body of retrospective epidemiologic knowledge that can be useful for the individual. The following discussion is a rather comprehensive presentation of the available data.

Burnell R. Brown, Jr.

During the past 30 years there has been a constant increase in the number of poor risk patients undergoing surgery and anesthesia for both emergency and elective surgical procedures. This has increased the number of patients anesthetized who have arteriosclerotic, hypertensive, and other forms of heart disease common in the older patient. This increase, in part at least, reflects merely the rapid rise in the population of the number of persons past 50 years of age. These geriatric patients have posed many problems for the anesthesiologist, not the least of which has been the evaluation of the patient's ability to withstand the stresses of anesthesia and surgery.

Studies have been undertaken to evaluate the patient who has suffered a myocardial infarction and to ascertain the operative or postoperative recurrence rate. An investigation attempting to determine factors affecting recurrence of infarction was reported in 1962 by me and others at Cornell Medical College; 35,937 consecutive patients were evaluated during the years 1959 to 1962.[1] Only cases of coronary occlusion proven by electrocardiogram or eventual postmortem examination were included for statistical analysis. The study was made to determine whether or not the time interval between the previous myocardial infarction and surgery and anesthesia had an effect on the recurrence rate (Table 1).

Since it was noted that 80 percent of the patients who had suffered a preoperative infarct were males over 50 years of age,

Table 1. Incidence of Postoperative Coronary Occlusions in the Male Surgical Population Over 50 Years of Age.

		No Post-operative Coronary Occlusion	Post-operative Coronary Occlusion
No previous history of coronary occlusion	8557	8498	59(0.7%)
Previous history of coronary occlusion	427	401	26(6%)

(Knapp, R. B., Topkins, M. J., and Artusio, J. F.: *The cerebrovascular accident and coronary occlusion in anesthesia.* J.A.M.A. 182:332, 1962. Copyright, 1962, American Medical Association.)

ANESTHESIA AND THE PATIENT WITH HEART DISEASE

this group was selected for detailed evaluation. Of the 8984 males, 8557 had no previous history of myocardial infarction, while 427 did—an incidence of 4.75 percent. Of the 8557 patients with no previous history, 59 demonstrated a postoperative myocardial infarction—an incidence of 0.7 percent. Of the 427 patients with a previous history of infarction, 26, or 6 percent, demonstrated a postoperative myocardial infarction.

Of the 59 patients with no previous history of myocardial infarction who suffered a postoperative infarct, 11 died—an incidence of mortality of 19 percent (Table 2). Of the 26 who had both a preoperative and postoperative myocardial infarction, 15 died—an incidence of 58 percent.

All 26 patients suffering a recurrent myocardial infarct postoperatively had their previous insult within 3 years of surgery; 89 percent had their previous infarct within 20 months of surgery (23 of 26 patients). The overall incidence of coronary occlusion in the male population over 50 years of age is approximately 1 percent.[2] In the surgical population in this study, the incidence was 4.75 percent (427 of 8984).

This study indicated that the incidence of recurrence of infarction following surgery was definitely diminished if the occlusion occurred 2 years or more prior to surgery.

Table 2. Mortality from Postoperative Coronary Occlusion in the Male Surgical Population Over 50 Years of Age.

		Post-operative Coronary Occlusion	Mortality from Post-operative Coronary Occlusion
No previous history of coronary occlusion	8557	59	11(19%)
Previous history of coronary occlusion	427	26	15(58%)

(Knapp, R. B., Topkins, M. J., and Artusio, J. F.: *The cerebrovascular accident and coronary occlusion in anesthesia.* J.A.M.A. 182:332, 1962. Copyright, 1962, American Medical Association.)

Statistical analysis failed to indicate that the type of anesthesia, the anesthetic agent, or the nature of the surgery played a role in recurrence of infarction.

The Cornell study was extended for a 5-year period by Topkins and Artusio.[3] The number of investigated male surgical patients over age 50 increased from 8,984 to 12,712. Of the 12,504 patients with no previous history of a myocardial infarction, 79 sustained a postoperative infarct—an incidence of 0.66 percent. Of the 658 patients with a preoperative infarction, 43 sustained one postoperatively, for an occurrence rate of 6.5 percent. Thus, the incidence is 10 times greater for patients with a preoperative infarction than for those without.

The mortality rate from postoperative infarction in patients with no previous history of infarction was 26.5 percent, as compared with 70 percent for patients with such a history.

In those with an infarct within 6 months of surgery, the recurrence rate was 54.5 percent. Between 6 months and 2 years, the incidence ranged between 20 percent and 25 percent. After 2 years, the rate dropped sharply to 5.9 percent. In this study, with a larger group of patients than in my previous investigation, the incidence of infarction was 5.2 percent, as compared with 4.75 percent in the earlier study and 1 percent in the population at large for males over 50.

From analysis of both Cornell studies, it is apparent that the danger of recurrence of infarction is during the first 6 months following myocardial infarction. After 3 years the recurrence rate of 1 percent equals the rate in males over 50 in the general population who have never undergone a previous infarction. However, it appears that the mortality rate following postoperative infarctions is independent of the time interval between preoperative infarction and surgery.

In June 1978, Steen and coworkers from the Mayo Clinic also reported an investigation of reinfarction after anesthesia and surgery.[4] They studied 587 patients with verified previous myocardial infarctions who were undergoing surgery, excluding cardiac procedures. Thirty-six patients (6.1 percent) experienced reinfarction within 7 days of surgery. Twenty-five of these thirty-six patients died (69 percent). Of the 15 patients who had suffered a myocardial infarction less than 3 months previously, postoperative reinfarction occurred in 4 (27 percent). The reinfarction rate in patients having surgery 6 months or more after the myocardial infarction stabilized at 4 percent to 5 percent.

There was no significant difference in the reinfarction rate between the sexes (6 percent for men and 6.6 percent for women). The reinfarction rate showed a trend toward an increase with age for patients older than 40 years.

Patients with preoperative hypertension had a greater risk of reinfarction than normotensive patients. The reinfarction rate was 9.4 percent in the hypertensive patients, which was significantly different from the 4.7 percent rate in nonhypertensive patients. This difference in rate is not true for diabetics versus nondiabetics, or for those with or without angina. The site of previous infarction played no role in reinfarction rate or in mortality. As in the previous Cornell studies, no differences in reinfarction rates were found for the different anesthetic techniques or agents.

The rate of recurrence in this study, however, was significantly higher in patients having intrathoracic and upper abdominal surgery, as compared with surgery at other sites. The reinfarction rate increased with the duration of anesthesia, from 5.9 percent for procedures lasting less than 3 hours to 15.9 percent for those lasting longer than 3 hours. It is interesting to note that in this study there was no difference in mortality between those admitted to an intensive care unit postoperatively and those not admitted or admitted after the diagnosis of reinfarction was made.

In agreement with the two Cornell investigations, it was apparent that the risk of a new myocardial infarction diminished after a 6-month interval. One conclusion, not previously reported, was that the incidence of reinfarction doubled if patients had pre-existing hypertension.

Intraoperative hypotension was associated with a higher reinfarction rate (15.2 percent versus 3.2 percent in patients without hypotensive episodes). Of course, the intraoperative hypotensive episode could be either the cause or the result of a reinfarction. Determination of cause versus effect was not made in this study.

The increase in repeated myocardial infarctions with increasing duration of anesthesia could well be due to the fact that the mean duration was longer for thoracic and upper abdominal surgery groups. As in the Cornell studies, mortality from reinfarctions was high (69 percent). Contributing factors are the added stress of surgery, anesthetics, and surgical pain in a patient experiencing a second myocardial infarction.

A study by Goldman and coworkers from the Massachusetts General Hospital in 1977 attempted to determine which preoperative factors might affect the development of cardiac complications after major noncardiac operations.[2] The investigators studied 1001 patients over 40 years of age. Of 58 patients manifesting postoperative cardiac complications, 19 died; 18 of the 58 patients developed documented intraoperative or postoperative myocardial infarctions. Analysis identified nine preoperative variables that had statistically significant correlation with life-threatening or fatal cardiac complications. Each of these variables was assigned points, derived by arriving at a discriminate function coefficient and dividing each coefficient by 0.05. The variables and their points were as follows:

1. S_3 gallop or distention of the jugular vein (11)
2. Myocardial infarction within the preceding 6 months (10)
3. Other than sinus rhythm (including premature atrial contractions) on the electrocardiogram (7)
4. More than five premature ventricular extra systoles at any time prior to surgery (7)
5. Intraperitoneal, intrathoracic, or aortic procedures (3)
6. Age greater than 70 (5)
7. Aortic stenosis (3)
8. Emergency surgery (4)
9. Poor general medical condition, including preoperative hypoxemia, hypokalemia, acidosis, chronic liver disease, or being bedridden by noncardiac causes (3)

Using these coefficients, 81 percent of the cardiac outcomes were correctly classified. A total of 53 points are possible, and three categories of patients have been classified by point value. Those with 5 points or less had an incidence of cardiac mortality of 0.2 percent; those with 6 to 25 points had a mortality of 2 percent; and those with greater than 25 points had a cardiac mortality of 56 percent.

The authors agreed with the conclusion that elective surgical procedures should be postponed for at least 6 months after an infarction. They claim that, by application of the multifactorial index, even patients with recent preoperative infarctions can be separated into high risk and low risk subgroups. Goldman and coworkers consider premature ventricular contractions important, largely because they are an indication of more severe heart disease.

Premature atrial contractions are usually regarded as benign, but in this study they sometimes indicated marginal cardiac reserve. The investigators recommend that only life-saving procedures be performed on patients with risk index scores of 26 points or more. Patients with index scores of 13 to 25 points have a sufficient cardiac risk to warrant preoperative cardiac consultation and a delay of surgery until the patient is medically more stable.

Conclusions that can be reached from the four studies described are:
1. Elective surgery should be deferred for at least 6 months following a documented myocardial infarct
2. The choice of anesthetic or anesthetic technique plays no significant role in the incidence of recurrence of an infarction
3. Strong statistical evidence implicates the thorax and upper abdomen as surgical sites that increase risk of infarction
4. Procedures lasting longer than 3 hours have a much higher risk than those of shorter duration
5. Nine preoperative factors affect the development of cardiac complications postoperatively, and, if several of these are present concurrently, surgery should be deferred until the cardiac problems are stabilized

REFERENCES

1. Knapp, R.B., Topkins, M.J., and Artusio, J.F.: *The cerebrovascular accident and coronary occlusion in anesthesia.* J.A.M.A. 182:332, 1962.
2. Goldman, M.D., et al.: *Multifactorial index of cardiac risk in noncardiac surgical procedures.* N. Engl. J. Med. 294:845, 1977.
3. Topkins, M.J., and Artusio, J.F.: *Myocardial infarction and surgery, a five year study.* Anesth. Analg. (Cleve.) 23:716, 1964.
4. Steen, P.A., Tinker, J.H., and Tarhan, S.: *Myocardial reinfarction after anesthesia and surgery.* J.A.M.A. 239:2655, 1978.

ANESTHESIA FOR PATIENTS WITH ISCHEMIC HEART DISEASE*

John H. Tinker, M.D.

An everyday happening in the life of anesthetists is the discovery that a patient scheduled for a noncardiac procedure has coronary artery disease. What should be done by the anesthetic consultant? What constitutes a "go" or "no go" situation? What anesthetic technique and monitoring systems should be employed? What is the risk to the patient? These are pragmatic questions answered in the light of presently available documentation by Dr. Tinker's article. His style is extremely lucid and makes for pleasant, informative reading. An excellent reference list on the state of the art in these clinical situations has been compiled by Dr. Tinker.

Burnell R. Brown, Jr.

*Supported in part by Grant NIH GM 24531 from the National Institutes of Health.

An estimated 675,000 people in the United States die each year from ischemic heart disease and related complications. About 1.3 million Americans suffer myocardial infarction each year, more than 0.5 percent of the entire U.S. population.[1] At least 4 million people in this country have clinically evident coronary artery disease (angina and/or prior infarct). Perhaps 10 times more have asymptomatic disease.[2] We hope that recent advances regarding protection of the potentially ischemic myocardium, reduction of infarct size, and care of acute myocardial infarctions have improved this grim picture. Realistically, there is little evidence that this improvement, if any, is very great. A recent repeat[3] of a decade-old study[4] of perioperative myocardial infarction (MI) did not show statistically significant improvement in either incidence or mortality. The early, relatively uncontrolled, enthusiastic reports [5-7] of coronary artery bypass grafting (CABG) are being supplanted by more sobering (perhaps better controlled) results.[8] Preston[9] states, "The history of medical therapeutics is that most treatments do not stand the test of time, especially those which are controversial within the profession itself." Most "treatment" and "prevention" of coronary artery disease (CAD) is controversial.

On a typical operating schedule there will often be a patient who has suffered a prior MI. Someone will suffer enough angina or hypertension, or both, to be taking propranolol. There also will likely be someone with a long history of congestive failure taking digitalis. This chapter will attempt to give a practical approach to anesthetic management for these patients. They often question their anesthesiologist about risk, and this chapter will explore that question. Two other areas of general interest will be included, namely, a brief history of therapeutic attempts at alleviating CAD and a discussion of methods of protection (practical and laboratory) of the ischemic myocardium.

HISTORY OF THERAPY FOR CAD

Nonsurgical therapy of CAD has generally been limited to symptomatic treatment. Angina pectoris has only one known cause, namely, an ischemic myocardium. The use of nitroglycerin to dilate capacitance vessels and decrease myocardial oxygen demand, and the development of beta-adrenergic blockade to decrease myocardial response to sympathetic stimulation both really constitute symptomatic therapy of CAD. The medical story also includes development of coronary intensive care units, with extensive beat-to-beat monitoring for arrhythmias, and burgeoning knowledge of mechanisms of arrhythmia generation and pharmacologic therapy. These are also symptomatic treatments. There are no agents to dissolve atherosclerotic plaques and no drugs that dramatically shift blood flow to infarcting areas; nor is there precise delineation of the initial mechanisms of intimal injury that result much later in the formation of an atherosclerotic lesion.

The surgical history of therapy for CAD is perhaps of more interest in its detail to anesthesiologists, especially with today's enthusiasm for coronary artery bypass grafting (CABG). Sympathectomy for angina was proposed in 1899,[10] although the procedure itself was not reported performed until the work of Jonnesco[11] in 1920. Jonnesco's patient reported superb pain relief, as have many thousands since, following various operations. By 1927, Cutler reported that about 75 percent of patients could expect significant angina relief from one or another denervation procedure.[12] Lindgren[13] reported 105 such procedures (with an 8.5 percent surgical mortality) with at least 80 percent pain relief. Cardiac denervations of various sorts were being performed until the late 1960s, when coronary bypass procedures appeared. Enthusiasm waned for these approaches, largely with the realization that many anatomically different procedures led to similar pain relief, which was often short-lived. Harken and coworkers[14] and Ellis and associates[15] concluded that although painful impulses arising in ischemic myocardium do pass through sectionable nerves, operations should be designed to increase myocardial blood supply. Preston[16] estimates that 1000 to 3000 cardiac denervation operations were done over 50 years, with operative mortality averaging about 10 percent.

The major surgical thrust, starting with the work of Claude Beck, has been to try to increase myocardial blood flow. Beck[17] created epicardial inflammation, stimulating adhesions and additional blood supply. This was accomplished in numerous procedures with sand, talc, magnesium silicate, and even asbestos, as well as with grafts of many abdominal and thoracic tissues. Operative mortality was 50 percent in Beck's 1937 report,[18] but the survivors either experienced superb relief of angina or were afraid to say otherwise. Despite the inevitable controversy over the Beck approach, about 2000 such procedures were performed over 25 years, with an estimated operative mortality of 15 percent.[19] Coronary sinus occlusion was tried in 1939[20] and was eventually added to the Beck procedure.[21] The curious idea behind this approach was that, although coronary blood flow decreased, anastomotic channels might be recruited by increased venous pressure.

The "logical" next step was to force arterial blood into the coronary sinus via a vein graft from the aorta, followed two months later by distal ligations of the coronary sinus (the graft tore if the procedures were done together).[22] Did these attempts at increasing myocardial blood flow actually decrease mortality? Beck[23] reported a comparison between a surgical group of 137 patients (a 2-year mortality rate of 13 percent) and a "medical" group (a 2-year mortality rate of 30 percent) in a pioneering study that recognized the need for (and encountered the difficulties of) such a comparison. All too often, however, the dictum was "one cannot deny anyone the obvious benefits of this logical operation just to have a control group."

Because of an earlier demonstration of remote anatomic connections between internal mammary and coronary arteries,[24] ligation of the internal mammaries was tried. Battezati and associates[25] reported 304 such operations in 1959, with 90 percent symptomatic relief of angina and 64 percent electrocardiographic improvement. Experiments in laboratory animals did not support this easily performed operation.[26] It had sufficiently low morbidity that controlled "blinded" studies were possible, and the famous "sham" operations, simulating internal mammary ligations, were performed by Cobb and coworkers[27] and Dimond and associates.[28] In both studies, the sham operation led to equal or better pain relief.

The next chapter in the history of surgery for CAD belongs to the Vineberg procedure,[29] that of implanting a bleeding internal mammary artery into a tunnel created by a blunt rod or clamp in the left ventricular wall. Preston[30] calls this procedure, when first viewed, "akin to spearing the heart in a sterile ambience." An entire cardiology residency of arrhythmias could cross the oscilloscope during the stormy postoperative course. Whether the procedure eventually did any good or not, no one argued that the first few postoperative hours and days were difficult. Other surgeons took up the procedure after a demonstration that connections had developed between the implant and the coronary arterial tree in two patients whose implants had been performed 5 and 7 years earlier.[31] Sewell[32] in 1972 reported a statistically significant reduction in mortality utilizing a life-table analysis following the Vineberg procedure. Perhaps 15,000 to 20,000 such procedures have been done.

Did anyone attack the coronaries themselves during these years? Bailey and coworkers[33] reported a survivor after coronary endarterectomy in 1957, but high mortality rates soon followed. Sawyer and associates[34] tried gas endarterectomies to dissect coronary lesions, but again with high risk.

Direct arterial anastomosis, pioneered in dogs in 1954 by Murray and coworkers,[35] was first done in man in the now-familiar form of aorta-to-coronary saphenous vein bypass by Favaloro and associates[36] and Johnson and coworkers[37] in 1969. Dozens of reports, totaling many thousands of cases, have been published regarding this operation to date, with high controversy as more and more "controls" have been applied. The obvious economic effects of CABG have been noticed by surgeons (favorably), internists (unfavorably), and government. Criticism in the lay press by leading surgeons of relatively unfavorable recent studies has tended to be vociferous but anecdotal.

Why go to this length to describe the history of medicine's attack on a common problem in a text on anesthesia? Today's students, exposed to these historical approaches to coronary artery disease, are filled with disbelief that such approaches were inflicted upon patients. Yet initial results of each type of procedure were uniformly "excellent." There is always a desire for positive results, fueled, perhaps, by many journals' ready acceptance of the reports. There is also a tendency to accept common disease and to focus on rarity or unusual forms. Truth to tell, spectacular progress is not evident in understanding this extremely common disease. Today's coronary artery bypass graft may be viewed with similar derision in the future.

The interested reader is referred to the excellent recent treatise by Preston,[2] from which much of the preceding information is condensed.

RISK

In the preoperative visit the anesthesiologist seldom refers to risk. When asked, "What is the risk of a general anesthetic?" we often respond with flippancies, such as "It is less than the risk of driving to the hospital." Patients are entitled to better information than this if they ask and if it exists.

Tarhan and associates[4] described in detail the significant risk of reinfarction occurring within 7 days of operation in patients who had suffered previous MI. In a study of more than 32,000 cases of anesthetics administered during 1967 and 1968, they reported a 0.13 percent incidence of MI if there was no previous MI, compared with a 6 percent overall incidence of new MI in patients with prior MI. If that prior MI was less than 3 months old at the time of surgery, the incidence of reinfarction was 37 percent, decreasing to 16 percent if the prior MI was 3 to 6 months old, and leveling off at 6 percent thereafter. Mortality from these perioperative reinfarctions was distressingly high at 50 percent.

Because enflurane, neuroleptanesthesia, and propranolol came into wide use after that study, and because ICU admissions following surgery had presumably increased in those high-risk patients, we repeated the study in patients anesthetized at the same institution during 1974 and 1975.[3] We were also interested in whether or not increased awareness of the problem might itself lead to improvement. During 1974 and 1975, 73,321 patients underwent anesthesia and noncardiac surgery, of whom 587 had suffered prior MI. If the patient's prior MI was less than 3 months old, the incidence of reinfarction was 27 percent; if the old MI had occurred 3 to 6 months previously, 11 percent suffered a new MI; and again, the overall incidence of reinfarction was 5 percent to 6 percent. None of these numerical decreases in incidence from the previous study were statistically significant. Worse, the mortality rate was (numerically) higher at 69 percent.[3]

In addition, angina, hypertension, and diabetes were examined as risk factors in patients with prior MI who were undergoing anesthesia and surgery. Preoperative hypertension, but not the others, could be statistically shown to be associated with increased risk of reinfarction. Enflurane was the most commonly employed volatile agent, but no anesthetic technique was associated with statistically increased or decreased risk. Intraoperative hypotension, defined as a 30 percent decrease in systolic blood pressure for one or more periods of at least 10 minutes, was associated with a significantly higher reinfarction rate, whereas intraoperative hypertension (defined as a similar increase) was not.

Operations on the thorax, upper abdomen, or great vessels were associated with incidences of reinfarction higher than those of the overall group. There was also a strikingly positive correlation between anesthesia time and reinfarction incidence. Admission to an ICU was not routine just because of prior MI. Whether or not the patient was admitted to an ICU for other reasons following surgery affected neither the incidence nor the outcome of reinfarctions. Retrospective studies, with all their limitations, do perhaps "tell it like it is." This study, though possibly not indicative of results obtainable by state-of-the-art prospective treatment, seems an indication that perioperative management of patients with CAD in a busy clinical setting still permits a relatively high incidence of MI, with a very high mortality rate.

Many patients with prior CABG will require subsequent noncardiac operations. In a recent study, Mahar and coworkers[38] examined the risk of anesthesia and noncardiac surgery in 99 patients with prior CABG who underwent 168 subsequent operations. This group was compared with a group of 49 patients who had angiographic evidence of CAD (greater than 50 percent stenosis of one or more major coronary arteries), who did not undergo CABG, but who then had noncardiac surgery. The group with CAD without CABG had the expected 6 percent incidence of perioperative MI. All patients in this group who suffered perioperative MI had three-vessel CAD. Thus, three-vessel CAD appears to be a risk factor similar in importance to prior MI. In the group of patients who had first undergone CABG, there were no MIs following 168 noncardiac operations. The difference between the two groups was statistically significant. The groups were not perfectly comparable because of the intervening CABG in one group. Still, the CABG group had angiographically worse CAD than did the non-CABG group. Whether this is evidence that CABG is efficacious is arguable, but the study does indicate that the risk of anesthesia and noncardiac surgery in patients with prior CABG is relatively low. Two other studies (without comparisons to medical groups) are in agreement.[39, 40]

Recommendations for the clinical anesthesiologist, based on the preceding risk data, are as follows. Elective anesthesia and surgery within 6 months of MI is still contraindicated. Patients with prior MI, combined with hypertension, are at greater risk, as are those scheduled for thoracotomy, upper abdominal surgery, and operations on the great vessels. The famous medicalservice transfer note that says "don't let the blood pressure fall" is statistically valid in patients with prior MI. Finally, operations on patients who have survived CABG are probably less risky than those on patients with prior MI or three-vessel CAD.

PREOPERATIVE EVALUATION

There are three areas of special interest in evaluating patients with CAD. First, it would be ideal to ascertain the patient's maximum ability to deliver oxygen to potentially ischemic myocardial areas, i.e., to completely assess regional myocardial perfusion. Second, it would be ideal to obtain a basal measure of the patient's myocardial contractility, coupled with measurement of how much that contractility can be increased by endogenous sympathetic stimulation (cardiac reserve). Third, any cardiovascular drugs the patient might be taking are of concern.

Myocardial Perfusion

Even with coronary angiography plus radionuclide scintigraphy, it is not possible to precisely delineate human regional myocardial perfusion. A prior myocardial infarct gives little information as to which, if any, area of myocardium is "next in line" for ischemia. The usual preoperative resting ECG is woefully inadequate in this regard. It is surprising how often we take comfort in the "normal" resting ECG as evidence that no significant CAD is present. The exercise test is much better; a negative exercise ECG indicates reasonably adequate coronary circulation and simulates the sympathetic stimulation that may accompany operation. A patient with angina or prior MI should at least undergo exercise electrocardiographic testing prior to elective surgery. History of exercise tolerance, carefully elicited, is also useful. Angina is the most reliable symptom of inadequate regional myocardial perfusion. Details of angina, including how much nitroglycerin is being used, whether use is increasing, and what exercise brings it about, should be obtained. Patients desiring other than CABG surgery may deny angina. A patient with a healed MI who has angina clearly has another compromised area of myocardium, and the mortality rate with a perioperative reinfarction is at least 50 percent. Because there is evidence that coronary artery bypass grafting reduces mortality, at least when left main coronary disease is present, consideration of this operation prior to other elective surgery may be advisable.[8] If a single significant lesion not of the left main artery is present, current evidence does not indicate prophylactic CABG prior to other surgery.

Contractility

The second preoperative consideration, contractility, is also crucial to anesthetic management. Patients with severe CAD, prior infarcts, or ventricular aneurysms may have poor overall contractility. There are dozens of confusing and conflicting methods of assessing contractility. If biplanar left ventriculograms have been obtained, then ejection fraction can be calculated:

$$\frac{LV\ end\text{-}diastolic\ volume\ -\ LV\ end\text{-}systolic\ volume}{LV\ end\text{-}diastolic\ volume}$$

Vlietstra and coworkers[41] have shown prospectively that ejection fraction is a valid predictor of 2- to 3-year outcome with and without CABG. Patients with ejection fractions of 25 to 50 percent had significantly better outcomes (2-year follow-up) following CABG than if treated medically. When ejection fractions were less than 25 percent, patients did poorly whether in the medical or surgical groups. Those with ejection fractions of 50 percent or more did equivalently well. A low ejection fraction (less than 50 percent) indicates a patient who likely will not easily tolerate negative inotropic drugs. Without sophisticated estimates of contractility, again history of exercise tolerance is an index of contractility. Fluoroscopic assessment of cardiac motion is notoriously subjective. Ejection fraction can also be estimated by echocardiography.

Drug Therapy

Finally, what about the patient's drug therapy? In general, drugs required preoperatively are still needed during anesthesia. This most emphatically *includes* propranolol. To rob the heart of its ability to respond to the stress of anesthesia and surgery, once taboo, is also to reduce the heart's ability to outstrip its (inadequate) regional blood supply. Because the normal heart can increase resting output five or six times, and because myocardial tissue is often normal in CAD, demand for O_2 in compromised regions can soon outstrip supply. Propranolol relieves angina by rendering normal heart muscle less able to increase O_2 demand, conserving the relatively limited supply. Angina, warning of such a deadly regional imbalance of O_2 supply and demand, is obliterated during anesthesia. Continued partial beta-adrenergic blockade is reasonable to insure against development of this imbalance. Kaplan and associates[42] have shown that continuing propranolol preoperatively does not result in increased morbidity or mortality during anesthesia and cardiac surgery. This blunts earlier warnings that beta-adrenergic blocked patients would not stand the stress of anesthesia.

Active patients may require large doses of propranolol for control of angina. These patients often tolerate modest preoperative reduction of dosage, especially if they are essentially at bed rest a few days prior to surgery. This will allow increased tolerance of negative inotropic drugs (anesthetics) intraoperatively. Propranolol should never be stopped abruptly. If angina returns during gradual reduction of dosage, a return toward the former dosage should again eliminate angina before elective anesthesia and surgery. Patients with angina despite enough propranolol to yield hemodynamic changes at low activity levels (e.g., postural hypotension, low exercise tolerance) should undergo angiography and be considered for CABG. Patients having angina the night before or morning of elective surgery must have developing MI ruled out before proceeding.

Digitalis is the other cardiovascular drug of concern to anesthesiologists. Many digitalized patients are also taking diuretics that cause loss of potassium and are likely potassium-depleted. Digitalis, diuretics, intraoperative electrolytic shifts caused by hypocarbia, iatrogenic administration of water, plus enhancement of arrhythmias by anesthetics have led many to recommend stopping digitalis one half-life prior to major surgery (e.g., 36 to 48 hours for digoxin). We would discontinue digitalis prior to major abdominal, vascular, cardiac, and thoracic surgery, but probably not do so prior to surgery in which less major physiologic disruption is expected. We would not, for example, stop digoxin prior to total hip replacement, unless evidence of digitalis toxicity was present. To indicate the range of opinion on this subject: prophylactic digitalization prior to surgery in older patients has been advocated.[43]

In this context is the problem of the patient with borderline low serum K^+, who is taking digitalis and scheduled for surgery tomorrow. The answer is *not* to run 80 mEq of KCl into the patient by vein overnight and measure another serum K^+ just as the infusion is finished! Clearly, all or very nearly all this KCl will be rapidly excreted. It is best to postpone surgery and re-establish K^+ stores orally, a process requiring several weeks. The common "solution" mentioned previously, while it does little to total body K^+, may temporarily increase *extracellular* K^+, which may protect the patient against digitalis-anesthetic-induced arrhythmias. The author, faced with such a patient whose surgery is urgent, would induce anesthesia with a slow infusion of KCl running at approximately 10 to 15 mEq/hour, avoid halothane, and consider an infusion of lidocaine at the earliest sign of trouble. If the serum $K^+ = 3.0$, do you cancel? What about 2.5? The latter should be postponed. A K^+ of 3.0 would seem marginally acceptable for proceeding in such a patient, if digitalis toxicity is not present.

Premedication for the patient with CAD should be relatively heavy. These patients may be harmed by anxiety-induced catecholamine release, occurring during procedures and examinations when the patients are awake. Narcotic premedication might obtund angina, thereby excluding a valuable symptom. The patient should be permitted nitroglycerin *ad lib,* and that drug should be carried by him to the operating room. Atropine I. M. does not increase heart rate enough to upset O_2 supply and demand, but it may not be needed as an antisialagogue with modern anesthetics. The author's preference for premedication is 10 to 30 mg diazepam P.O. with a sip of water 2 to 3 hours prior to surgery.

INTRAOPERATIVE MANAGEMENT

The patient with severe CAD, who is anxious already, may be caused more harm than benefit by painful and scary procedures performed "under local" while awake. Elevated heart rate or arterial pressure caused by sympathetic stimulation may lead to development of ischemic myocardium. Minute-to-minute measurement of blood pressure can be achieved with the traditional cuff. Patients with severe CAD do not automatically need arterial lines placed while they are awake. It may be worse to place the awake patient in steep Trendelenburg's position and insert a pulmonary artery or central venous pressure catheter.

Induction of anesthesia must be smooth, without large fluctuations in heart rate and blood pressure. Electrocardiographic monitoring should be by V_5 lead primarily, so as to best watch for ST segment depression (akin to an angina attack). Once electrocardiographic leads and one intravenous needle are in place, a careful induction with 100-mg increments of thiopental or 10-mg increments of diazepam is carried out until loss of eyelid reflex occurs. Unless the patient is critically ill, we would prefer to await loss of awareness before inserting arterial, central venous pressure, or pulmonary artery lines.

Three subjects must be discussed before continuing with clinical management: volatile agents, relaxants, and monitoring. Volatile agents (today, essentially halothane and enflurane) are negative inotropic drugs, to be sure, but they concomitantly depress overall myocardial oxygen consumption ($M\dot{V}o_2$). Whether or not decreasing O_2 consumption of normal myocardium protects potentially ischemic areas is controversial. Halothane-induced decreases in MVo_2 have been reported to decrease the size of experimental myocardial infarcts.[44] Still, excessive negative inotropic effect may lead to hypotension, with reduced coronary perfusion pressure. In potentially ischemic areas, because the diameter of vessels is relatively fixed, flow becomes dependent on pressure. Decreasing arterial pressure may lead to a vicious cycle: decreasing O_2 delivery leading to further ischemia, leading to less cardiac output, less arterial pressure, less O_2 delivery, and additional ischemia. Intraoperative hypotension has been associated with significantly higher reinfarction rates in patients with prior MI.[3] On the other hand, patients with CAD are often otherwise healthy. Unless sufficiently obtunded, surgically induced sympathetic stimulation may drive heart rate and arterial pressure to unacceptable levels.

Are there objective differences between the use of halothane and enflurane in these patients? One recent study, performed during trans-sphenoidal hypophysectomies in man, with large doses of epinephrine (and cocaine) applied to nasal mucosa, found that significantly fewer arrhythmias occurred with enflurane.[45] Arrhythmias are often considered benign by anesthesiologists. In fact they may increase average wall tension, limiting endocardial blood flow, and may signal the development of ischemia itself. We do not consider the development of any arrhythmia to be benign in patients with CAD. Nonetheless, halothane has been administered during millions of safe anesthetics. We think the question as to which anesthetic is best in patients with CAD has not been answered. Choice of anesthetic agent for a patient with CAD ideally should rest upon evidence of that agent's properties relative to CAD. Today, we seem to choose between agents for hepatic, renal, or even medicolegal reasons instead.

The large-dose narcotic techniques were intended for patients with severe low-output states, such as longstanding rheumatic mitral disease. Narcotics exert little myocardial depression, and the vasodilation acts as "internal phlebotomy." With CAD, however, the myocardium is often relatively normal. These vigorous patients may respond to narcotic/nitrous oxide anesthesia with unacceptable increases in heart rate and blood pressure.

Partial beta-adrenergic blockade, while clearly beneficial, nonetheless dictates reduction in dosage of volatile agents. This raises questions of awareness. An electrocardiographic shift, possibly indicative of loss of awareness, occurs at approximately 0.4 MAC with halothane, enflurane, and isoflurane in monkeys.[46] Anesthesiologists have long known that movement under anesthesia does not necessarily indicate awareness. These beta-blocked patients can often be given halothane or enflurane with N_2O totalling 0.5 to 1 MAC, achieving adequate amnesia and depression of sympathetic stimulation, without unacceptable hypotension.

Relaxants are the second management problem. Loeb and associates[47] have shown heart rate in man to be *much more* important as a determinant of development of myocardial ischemia than is systolic blood pressure. Therefore, the increase in heart rate caused by the vagolytic action of pancuronium is disturbing. Savarese and coworkers[48] have suggested metocurine as a possible substitute, reporting that it does not result in as much hypotension as *d*-tubocurarine. In the author's experience, 0.08 to 0.12 mg/kg pancuronium, given over 3 to 5 minutes following thiopental while ventilating the patient by mask with oxygen and volatile agent, does not result in worrisome increases in heart rate. Succinylcholine in most adults will not decrease heart rate enough for concern about hypotension or arrhythmias and is not contraindicated in patients with CAD.

ANESTHESIA FOR PATIENTS WITH ISCHEMIC HEART DISEASE   77

Finally, what does the clinician do about monitoring the patient with CAD? Much ado has recently been made of the "rate-pressure product." Multiplying heart rate by systolic arterial pressure has been correlated with $M\dot{V}o_2$ in humans. The problem is that monitoring overall $M\dot{V}o_2$ does not necessarily delineate oxygen delivery to the critical area(s). Loeb and associates[47] studied 20 patients with known CAD and angina. They deliberately increased $M\dot{V}o_2$ by 80 percent, using electrical pacing to heart rates of 140 beats per minute. Seventeen patients experienced angina, and fourteen had ischemic ST changes. After permitting $M\dot{V}o_2$ to return to control (awake) level, they again increased it to the same amount by increasing systolic pressure to about 190 torr, using methoxamine. This time only six patients experienced angina, and only three had ischemic ST changes. The difference was statistically significant at the same increases in overall $M\dot{V}o_2$. Thus, although rate-pressure product is a monitor of overall $M\dot{V}o_2$, we prefer *not* to multiply the two variables together. We concentrate especially upon not permitting large increases in heart rate.

Are arterial or pulmonary artery (PA) catheters needed for all patients with CAD? We think not, but we tend to place them for less major surgery in patients with CAD. Patients with CAD have primarily compromised left ventricles. Pulmonary capillary wedge pressures, reflecting left atrial pressures, which reflect left ventricular end-diastolic pressures, may not enable an immediate diagnosis of acute regional myocardial ischemia unless that ischemia is so massive as to begin to compromise overall ventricular function. A major vascular operation in a patient with CAD, in which significant blood loss is expected, would seem an example of a prime indication for a PA catheter.

To continue the discussion of routine management of intraoperative anesthesia, we have more or less justified the use of volatile agents. What about nitrous oxide? This almost ubiquitous agent is mildly negatively inotropic and reduces dosage of the volatile agent. Maroko and coworkers[49] demonstrated reduction of size in experimental infarcts by the use of 100 percent oxygen compared to 40 percent oxygen breathing in the dog. This logical idea is often overlooked in the operating room. Following intubation of the trachea in a patient with CAD, large increases in heart rate, which lead to depressed ST segments on the V-lead, are often treated with propranolol and increased concentrations of volatile agents. Seldom is the N_2O discontinued. The added PaO_2 does not greatly increase O_2 content, but studies, including one in man, have shown reduction in the size of infarcts by inhalation of oxygen-rich mixtures.[50]

Another oft-overlooked aspect of management in patients with CAD is temperature. Morris and coworkers[51] have shown that lightly anesthetized patients maintain body temperature satisfactorily only as long as operating room temperature is above 21°C (69°F); otherwise, gradual decreases in body temperature occur. Warming blankets in adults are of little value, because so little of the skin is in contact and because skin compressed by body weight is less able to exchange heat.[51] Hypothermic patients shiver violently upon awakening and have increases in whole body $\dot{V}O_2$ and excessive circulatory demands. The conditions of oxygen demand leading to postoperative infarctions may thus be initiated in the operating room. Scrupulous attention must be paid to the temperature of operating room air, plus that of irrigation, I.V. fluids, and sponges. The temperature in the operating room should be a prescription item, especially in patients with CAD.

What about blood gases? Can hypocarbia decrease coronary blood flow? Our usual mild hyperventilation has little effect on coronary flow, a circulation regulated largely by oxygen demand. Hemodynamic stability, no V-lead ST changes, no changes in ventilator settings, and no massive transfusions, for example, would seem to negate "routine" and expensive blood gases.

PROTECTION OF ISCHEMIC MYOCARDIUM

This subject has been recently reviewed.[1] For proper evaluation of any proposed therapy, it is necessary to quantitate the size of infarct. Epicardial artery ligation in a dog results in an obvious area of cyanosis within seconds. Epicardial and endocardial electrocardiographic leads from within this area show ST elevation promptly.[52] The ST segment will not elevate unless flow to that area has been reduced to about one third of control.[53] Unlike changes in transmural flow, reductions in subendocardial flow are not well reflected by epicardial (or precordial) ST changes.[54] In humans, extensive studies of various interventions using such "ST mapping" have been reported.[55, 56]

Ischemic myocardium releases enzymes, and there are numerous reports of measuring the size of infarcts by quantitating, with time, serial blood enzyme content. The disappearance of creatinine phosphokinase (CPK) is commonly utilized[57] and is reported to correlate with the size of infarct measured histologically at autopsy in man.[57, 58] About 7 hours (samples) are required before the curve of CPK disappearance can be accurately projected. Interventions can then be applied and studied, but irreversible damage may have already occurred.

Radionuclide myocardial imaging is gaining in popularity. It estimates the size of infarct by using cesium, potassium, rubidium, or thallium.[59-62] The resultant "cold spot" (area of poor or no perfusion) can be quantitated by combining biplanar projections. Comparing these scintigrams before and after exercise has also provided information on regional imbalance in supply and demand.[63] "Hot spot" imaging, using [99M]TC tetracycline, allows a positive picture of the infarcting area, for diagnosis of acute MI. One week after acute MI, the hot spot no longer is visible; thus, recent infarcts can be separated from old ones.[64]

Many investigators have used such estimates of the size of infarcts to determine if various interventions reduce or increase the size. Isoproterenol, with its well-known potent chronotropic effect, has been shown in several studies to increase the size of infarct after occlusion of the coronary artery.[65-69] The use of this agent is rarely justifiable in patients with CAD. Bradycardia with hypotension, often listed as an indication for isoproterenol, may already be due to myocardial ischemia. Isoproterenol may yield transient improvement, but with a larger resultant infarct. Digitalis in the nonfailing heart,[65] glucagon,[65, 69] bretylium tosylate,[65] tachycardia (pacer-induced),[65] and hyperthermia[70] have been shown to increase the size of experimental infarcts.

Propranolol leads the list of therapeutic interventions that have been shown to decrease the size of infarct in animals[71] and in man.[72] Scrutiny of the many papers reporting the benefits of beta-adrenergic blockade during acute MI is likely to result in increased use by anesthesiologists of propranolol during anesthesia and surgery for patients with CAD. Counterpulsation, digitalis in the failing heart, and even glucose-insulin-potassium (GIK) have reduced the size of infarct in man.[1] Bland and Lowenstein[44] have demonstrated reductions in size of infarct by decreasing $M\dot{V}O_2$ with halothane in dogs.

Nitroglycerin increases oxygen delivery to ischemic myocardium and reduces ST-segment evidence of injury, whereas both are worsened by nitroprusside given to decrease peripheral degrees of vascular resistance in man and animals.[73] Nitroprusside is probably contraindicated for reduction of afterload in patients with *actual* ischemic myocardium. With severe hypertension (some postoperative vascular cases, for example), nitroprusside would be reasonable, because an appropriate reduction in blood pressure (and ventricular wall tension) would make conversion of potentially ischemic myocardium into actually ischemic tissue less likely. Nitroglycerin for intravenous infusion is still not available. Because venodilation is so prominent an action, nitroglycerin is perhaps less effective than nitroprusside in decreasing afterload. Still, in patients with critical coronary artery lesions, the use of nitroprusside should be very cautious, indeed. Use of nitroprusside following coronary artery bypass grafting implies faith that the surgery has "revascularized" all important potentially ischemic areas. Nitroprusside has been recently reviewed.[74]

In the dog, large doses of corticosteroids significantly retard the healing of experimental myocardial infarcts.[75] Evidence regarding steroid-mediated reduction of the size of infarcts is not sufficiently convincing to constitute an indication for its use during anesthesia.[76]

Why are even small reductions in the size of infarcts so important? The heart has "extra" myocardium only in the sense that it is normally able to increase output greatly from that at rest. Reduction in viable myocardium results in limitation of that ability to increase output. In a most direct sense, "quality of life" is related to the heart's ability to meet whatever demands are placed upon it. Therefore, even small decreases in the size of infarcts, achieved through optimum care, whether during anesthesia or not, are critically important.

SUMMARY

The suggested anesthetic management of patients with potentially ischemic myocardium is as follows:
1. Careful work-up before proceeding if angina is present preoperatively.
2. Heavy premedication, attention to factors of preoperative

anxiety, and avoidance of unnecessary painful procedures in the awake patient. Do not stop propranolol.
3. Monitoring of ST segments via V_5 lead during anesthesia. Do not permit large fluctuations in systolic blood pressure or large increases in heart rate.
4. Maintenance of patient's temperature to obviate postoperative shivering.
5. Treatment of increased heart rate and ST segment changes with propranolol in 0.25-mg I.V. increments every 1 to 3 minutes until improvement noted (reasonable acute dose limit is 2 to 3 mg).
6. Treatment of ventricular arrhythmias with lidocaine bolus (50 to 100 mg) and infusion if more than one bolus is required (1 to 2 mg/70 kg/min), plus usual blood gases and electrolytes.

ACKNOWLEDGEMENT

The author wishes to thank Ms. Ann E. Tvedt for assistance in preparation of the manuscript.

REFERENCES

1. Hillis, L. D., and Braunwald, E.: *Myocardial ischemia* (3 parts). N. Engl. J. Med. 296:971, 1034, and 1093, 1977.
2. Preston, T. A.: *Coronary Artery Surgery: A Critical Review.* Raven Press, New York, 1977, p. 5.
3. Steen, P. A., Tinker, J. H., and Tarhan, S.: *Myocardial reinfarction after anesthesia and surgery.* J.A.M.A. 239:2566, 1978.
4. Tarhan, S., Moffitt, E. A., Taylor, W. F., et al.: *Myocardial infarction after general anesthesia.* J.A.M.A. 220:1451, 1972.
5. Sheldon, W. C., Rincon, G., Effler, D. B., et al.: *Vein graft surgery for coronary artery disease.* Circulation (Suppl. III) 48:184, 1973.
6. Mundth, E. D., and Austen, W. G.: *Surgical measures for coronary heart disease* (3 parts). N. Engl. J. Med. 293:13, 1975.
7. Cohn, L. H., Boyden, C. M., and Collins, J. J.: *Improved long-term survival after aortocoronary bypass for advanced coronary artery disease.* Am. J. Surg. 129:380, 1975.
8. Takaro, T., Hultgren, H. N., and Detre, K. M.: *VA cooperative study of coronary arterial surgery: II. Left main disease.* Circulation (Suppl. II) 52:143, 1975.
9. Preston, p. 7.
10. Francois-Franck, C. A.: *Signification physiologique de la resection*

du sympathetique dans la maladie de baseton, l'épilepsie, l'idistre, et la glaucome. Bull. Acad. Med. Paris 41:594, 1899.

11. Jonnesco T: *Traitement chirurgical de l'angine de poitrine guérie par la resection du sympathetique cervico-thoracique.* Bull. Acad. Med. Paris 84:93, 1920.

12. Cutler, E. C.: *The present status of the treatment of angina pectoris by cervical sympathectomy.* Ann. Clin. Med. 4:1004, 1927.

13. Lindgren, I.: *Angina Pectoris. A Clinical Study with Special Reference to Neurosurgical Treatment.* Ivar Haeggströms Boktryckeri, A. B., Stockholm, 1950.

14. Harken, D. E., Black, H., Dickson, J. F., et al.: *De-epicardialization: a simple, effective surgical treatment for angina pectoris.* Circulation 12:955, 1955.

15. Ellis, L. B., Blungart, H. L., Harken, D. E., et al.: *Long-term management of patients with coronary artery disease.* Circulation 17:945, 1958.

16. Preston, p. 9.

17. Beck, C. S.: *The development of a new blood supply to the heart by operation.* Ann. Surg. 102:801, 1935.

18. Beck, C. S.: *Coronary sclerosis and angina pectoris. Treatment by grafting a new blood supply upon the myocardium.* Surg. Gynecol. Obstet. 64:270, 1937.

19. Preston, p. 14.

20. Fauteux, M.: *Treatment of coronary disease with angina by pericoronary neurectomy combined with ligation of the great cardiac vein.* Am. Heart J. 31:260, 1946.

21. Beck, S. C., and Brofman, B. L.: *The surgical management of coronary artery disease: background, rationale, clinical experiences.* Ann. Intern. Med. 45:975, 1956.

22. Roberts, J. T., Browne, H. S., and Roberts, G.: *Nourishment of the myocardium by way of the coronary veins.* Fed. Proc. 2:90, 1943.

23. Beck, C. S.: *Coronary artery disease. A report to William Harvey 300 years later.* Am. J. Cardiol. 1:38, 1958.

24. Hudson,C. F., Moritz, A. R., and Wearn, J. T.: *The extracardiac anastomoses of the coronary arteries.* J. Exp. Med. 57:919, 1932.

25. Battezati, M., Tagliaferro, A., and Cattaneo, A. D.: *Clinical evaluation of bilateral internal mammary artery ligation as treatment of coronary heart disease.* Am. J. Cardiol. 4:180, 1959.

26. Sabiston, D. C., and Blalock, A.: *Experimental ligation of the internal mammary artery and its effect on coronary occlusion.* Surgery 43:906, 1958.

27. Cobb, L. A., Thomas, G. I., Dillard, D. H., et al.: *An evaluation of internal mammary artery ligation by a double blind technique.* N. Engl. J. Med. 260:115, 1959.

28. Dimond, E. G., Kittle, C. F., and Crockett, J. E.: *Comparison of inter-*

nal mammary artery ligation and sham operation for angina pectoris. Am. J. Cardiol, 5:483, 1960.

29. Vineberg, A., and Walker, J.: *Six months to six years experience with coronary artery insufficiency treated by internal mammary artery implantation.* Am. Heart J. 54:851, 1957.
30. Preston, p. 17.
31. Sones, F. M., and Shirey, E. K.: *Cine coronary arteriography.* Mod. Concepts Cardiovasc. Dis. 4:391, 1962.
32. Sewell, W. H.: *Life table analysis of the results of coronary surgery.* Chest 61:481, 1972.
33. Bailey, C. P., May, A., and Lemmon, W. M.: *Survival after coronary endarterectomy in man.* J.A.M.A. 164:641, 1957.
34. Sawyer, P. N., Kaplitt, M., Sobel, S., et al.: *Experimental and clinical experience with gas endarterectomy.* Arch. Surg. 95:736, 1967.
35. Murray, G., Porcheron, R., Hilario, J., et al.: *Anastomosis of a systemic artery to the coronary.* Can. Med. Assoc. J. 71:594, 1954.
36. Favaloro, R. G.: *Saphenous vein graft in the surgical treatment of coronary artery disease.* J. Thorac. Cardiovasc. Surg. 58:178, 1969.
37. Johnson, W. D., Flemma, R. J., Lepley, D., et al.: *Extended treatment of severe coronary artery disease: a total surgical approach.* Ann. Surg. 170:460, 1969.
38. Mahar, L. J., Steen, P. A., Tinker, J. H., et al.: *Perioperative myocardial infarction in patients with coronary artery disease with and without aorta-coronary artery bypass grafts.* J. Thorac. Cardiovasc. Surg. 76:533, 1978.
39. Scher, K. S., and Tice, D. A.: *Operative risks in patients with previous coronary artery bypass.* Arch. Surg. 111:807, 1976.
40. McCollum, C. H., Garcia-Rinaldi, R., Graham, J. M., et al.: *Myocardial revascularization prior to subsequent major surgery in patients with coronary artery disease.* Surgery 81:302, 1977.
41. Vlietstra, R. E., Assad-Morell, J. L., Frye, R. L., et al.: *Survival predictors in coronary artery disease: medical and surgical comparisons.* Mayo Clin. Proc. 52:85, 1977.
42. Kaplan, J. A., Dunbar, R. W., Bland, J. W., et al.: *Propranolol and cardiac surgery: a problem for the anesthesiologist?* Anesth. Analg. (Cleve.) 54:571, 1975.
43. Deutsch, S., and Dalen, J. E.: *Indications for prophylactic digitalization.* Anesthesiology 30:648, 1969.
44. Bland, J. H., and Lowenstein, E.: *Halothane-induced decrease in experimental myocardial ischemia in the non-failing canine heart.* Anesthesiology 45:287, 1976.
45. Horrigan, R. W., Eger, E. I., and Wilson, C.: *Nonlinear dose-response relationship of epinephrine induced ventricular irritability under enflurane anesthesia in man.* Proc. Am. Soc. Anesthesiol. Ann. Mtg. 1977, pp. 87–88.

46. Tinker, J. H., Sharbrough, F. W., and Michenfelder, J. D.: *Anterior shift of the dominant EEG rhythm during anesthesia in the Java monkey.* Anesthesiology 46:252, 1977.
47. Loeb, H. S., Sandje, A., Croke, R. P., et al.: *Effects of pharmacologically-induced hypertension on myocardial ischemia and coronary hemodynamics in patients with fixed coronary obstruction.* Circulation 57:41, 1978.
48. Savarese, J. J., Ali, H. H., and Antonio, R. P.: *The clinical pharmacology of metocurine: dimethyltubocurarine revisited.* Anesthesiology 47:277, 1977.
49. Maroko, P. R., Radvany, P., Braunwald, E., et al.: *Reduction of infarct size by oxygen inhalation following acute coronary occlusion.* Circulation 52:360, 1975.
50. Madias, J. E., Madias, N. E., and Hood, W. B.: *Precordial ST-segment mapping 2: effects of oxygen inhalation on ischemic injury in patients with acute myocardial infarction.* Circulation 53:411, 1976.
51. Morris, R. H., and Wilkey, B. R.: *The effects of ambient temperature on patient temperature during surgery not involving body cavities.* Anesthesiology 32:102, 1970.
52. Ross, J., Jr.: *Electrocardiographic ST-segment analysis in the characterization of myocardial ischemia and infarction.* Circulation (Suppl.I) 53:73, 1976.
53. Wegria, R., Segers, M., Keating, R. P., et al.: *Relationship between the reduction in coronary flow and the appearance of electrocardiographic changes.* Am. Heart J. 38:90, 1949.
54. Smith, H. J., Singh, B. N., Norris, R. M., et al.: *Changes in myocardial blood flow and ST-segment elevation following coronary artery occlusion in dogs.* Circ. Res. 36:697, 1975.
55. Braunwald, E., and Maroko, P. R.: *ST segment mapping: realistic and unrealistic expectations.* Circulation 54:529, 1976.
56. Hillis, L. D., Askenazi, J., Braunwald, E., et al.: *Use of changes in epicardial QRS complex to assess interventions which modify the extent of myocardial necrosis following coronary artery occlusion.* Circulation 54:591, 1976.
57. Shell, W. E., and Sobel, B. E.: *Biochemical markers of ischemic injury.* Circulation (Suppl. I) 53:98, 1976.
58. Bleifield, W. H., Haurath, P., and Mathey, D.: *Serial CPK determinations for evaluation of size and development of acute myocardial infarction.* Circulation (Suppl. I) 53:108, 1976.
59. Hurley, P. J., Cooper, M., Reba, R. C., et al.: *^{43}KCl: a new radiopharmaceutical for imaging the heart.* J. Nucl. Med. 12:516, 1971.
60. Romhilt, D. W., Adolph, R. J., Sodd, V. J., et al.: *Cesium-129 myocardial scintigraphy to detect myocardial infarction.* Circulation 48:1242, 1973.
61. Martin, N. D., Zaret, B. L., McGowan, R. L., et al.: *Rubidium-*

81: a new myocardial scanning agent. Radiology 111:651, 1974.

62. Strauss, H. W., Harrison, K., Langan, J. K., et al.: *Thallium-201 for myocardial imaging: relation of thallium-201 to myocardial perfusion. Circulation 51:641, 1975.*

63. Zaret, B. L., Strauss, H. W., Martin, N. D., et al.: *Noninvasive regional myocardial perfusion with radioactive potassium: a study of patients at rest, with exercise, and during angina pectoris.* N. Engl. J. Med. 288:809, 1973.

64. Zweiman, F. G., Holman, B. L., O'Keefe, A., et al.: *Selective uptake of* $^{99M\text{Tc}}$ *complexes and* ^{67}Ga *in acutely infarcted myocardium.* J. Nucl. Med. 16:975, 1975.

65. Maroko, P. R., Kjekshus, J. K., Sobel, B. E., et al.: *Factors influencing infarct size following experimental coronary artery occlusions.* Circulation 43:67, 1971.

66. Vatner, S. F., Millard, R. W., Patrick, T. A., et al.: *Effects of isoproterenol on regional myocardial function, electrogram, and blood flow in conscious dogs with myocardial ischemia.* J. Clin. Invest. 57:1261, 1976.

67. Mueller, H., Ayres, S. M., Gregory, J. J., et al.: *Hemodynamics, coronary blood flow, and myocardial metabolism in coronary shock; response to l-norepinephrine and isoproterenol.* J. Clin. Invest. 49:1885, 1970.

68. Maroko, P. R., Libby, P., Covell, J. E., et al.: *Precordial ST elevation mapping: an atraumatic method for assessing alterations in the extent of myocardial ischemic injury: effects of pharmacologic and hemodynamic interventions.* Am. J. Cardiol. 29:223, 1972.

69. Lekven, J., Kjekshus, J. K., and Mjös, O. D.: *Effects of glucagon and isoproterenol on severity of acute myocardial ischemic injury.* Scand. J. Clin. Lab. Invest. 32:129, 1973.

70. Liedtke, A. J., and Hughes, H. C.: *Hyperthermic insult to ischemic myocardium: implications of fever as an energy draining process in myocardial infarct.* Clin. Res. 24:227, 1976.

71. Gold, H. K., Leinbach, R. C., and Maroko, P. R.: *Propranolol-induced reduction of signs of ischemic injury during acute myocardial infarction.* Am. J. Cardiol. 38:689, 1976.

72. Mueller, H. S., Ayres, S. M., Religa, A., et al.: *Propranolol in the treatment of acute myocardial infarction.* Circulation 49:1078, 1974.

73. Chiariello, M., Gold, H. K., Leinbach, R. C., et al.: *Comparison between the effects of nitroprusside and nitroglycerin on ischemic injury during acute myocardial infarction.* Circulation 54:766, 1976.

74. Tinker, J. H., and Michenfelder, J. D.: *Sodium nitroprusside, pharmacology, toxicology and therapeutics.* Anesthesiology 45:340, 1976.

75. Green, R. M., Cohen, J., and DeWeese, J. A.: *Short term use of cor-*

ticosteroids after experimental myocardial infarction: effects on ventricular function and infarct healing. Circulation (Suppl. III) 50:103, 1974.

76. Roberts, R., de Mello, V., and Sobel, B. E.: *Deleterious effects of methylprednisolone in patients with myocardial infarction.* Circulation (Suppl. I) 53:204, 1976.

ANESTHETIC CONSIDERATIONS IN ESSENTIAL HYPERTENSION

Burnell R. Brown, Jr., M.D., Ph.D.

It has been estimated that 23 million adult Americans can be classified essential hypertensives—approximately 10 percent of the entire population. Most of these cases of hypertension are either not recognized or are inadequately treated, and the majority of them fit into the borderline or mild hypertensive group. Although data on anesthetic risks and pros and cons of various anesthetic regimens in the hypertensive patient are woefully lacking, there is sufficient consensus and clinical experience available to formulate guidelines. It is rather unusual that such a common disease, one responsible directly or indirectly for over 750,000 deaths per year, should be so incompletely studied insofar as anesthesia and surgery are concerned.

PATHOPHYSIOLOGY AND CLASSIFICATION OF HYPERTENSION

It is assumed in this chapter that secondary causes of hypertension, such as pheochromocytoma and aldosteronoma, have been ruled out and that the anesthesiologist is dealing exclusively with essential hypertension, a disease of unknown etiology defined as present when a casual diastolic blood pressure recording is 95 mm Hg or higher. The progression of the hypertensive state, from the asymptomatic individual with labile borderline elevations of diastolic blood pressure to the severe hypertensive with cardiac, renal, and neurologic disease, usually extends over a period of 15 to 20 years. In certain cases, however, the entire progression may be condensed into a very brief episode, as short as several months. This latter situation is defined as accelerated hypertension.

Borderline or Labile Hypertension

Borderline hypertension is defined by blood pressure readings of 150/90 to 160/100 mm Hg, interspersed with occasional normal determinations. There is no evidence of damage to target organs (e.g., heart, kidney, brain) at this stage. The cardiac output in borderline hypertension is frequently elevated; this phenomenon is more common in younger patients than in older, but the difference frequently disappears during stress tests. Propranolol will decrease this elevated cardiac output. Peripheral resistance in this stage is normal or very slightly elevated, and total blood volume may be low. The patient is usually asymptomatic.

Although long-term studies indicate that the mortality rate of these individuals is 1.4 to 2.7 times that of the normotensive population, there is little data to document that these patients are at higher risk than normotensive persons insofar as anesthesia is concerned. Clinical experience indicates that these patients may have a greater than usual drop in blood pressure when anesthetized with potent, halogenated, inhalation anesthetics. Although not proven, it can be speculated that this drop could be due to a reduction of the high cardiac output coupled with the low blood volume frequently attendant with early hypertension. On the other hand, the lability of blood pressure could produce "overshoot" to potentially harmful degrees of hypertension if a nitrous oxide-narcotic-relaxant sequence were employed.

Consensus indicates that these patients should be treated with antihypertensives and should be maintained on therapy. There is conclusive evidence that life span is increased by continuing appropriate therapy.

Mild Hypertension

This stage is also referred to as the phase of sustained elevation of diastolic pressure. Cardiac output is normal or slightly elevated, and there is a constant increase in total peripheral resistance. There may be early signs of cardiac failure, such as exercise dyspnea or nocturia. Optic fundi arteriovenous nicking may occur. There may be signs and symptoms of accelerated atherosclerosis. Essential hypertension and atherosclerosis are two different disease states, but hypertension certainly accelerates atherosclerotic changes. Thus, electrocardiographic findings may show slight evidence of left ventricular hypertrophy (a finding of hypertension), plus coronary atherosclerosis disease, such as conduction defects, ischemic alterations, and old infarctions.

Anesthetic mortality and morbidity in this phase is almost entirely due to atherosclerotic complications. If there are not significant laboratory signs or physical examination stigmata of atherosclerosis, the patient with essential hypertension in this phase is probably only a slightly higher risk than a healthy individual. He or she should be classified as an A.S.A. Class II patient.

Moderate Hypertension

This phase is defined by a diastolic blood pressure of 100 to 115 mm Hg at all times. Detectable damage to organs is usually present, particularly late in this phase, since the mean life span in this stage is approximately 6 years if the disease is untreated. All experts in the field agree that treatment in this phase is mandatory and life-saving. The untreated patient has a threefold higher rate of major complication than the treated. Treatment affords protection against stroke and congestive heart failure, but not against myocardial infarction, which is due to atherosclerosis.

Moderate to Severe Hypertension

This phase is defined by diastolic pressures of 115 to 130 mm Hg. These patients are at very high risk for major complications in a short period. In the V.A. Cooperative Hypertension Study, 30 percent of untreated patients at this phase developed complications within only 18 months. These patients represent a major anesthetic risk. The problems include cerebrovascular accidents, myocardial infarction, congestive heart failure, and renal decompensation. Adequate treatment prolongs life span. In addition, the cause of death is more related to atherosclerotic than hypertensive complications in treated patients. The leading causes of death in the untreated individual with severe hypertension, in order of frequency, are stroke, congestive heart failure, myocardial infarction, and renal failure. In treated hypertensives, myocardial infarction is the leading cause of death. These patients represent A.S.A. Class III.

CLINICAL QUESTIONS

With this basic background on hypertension, the remainder of this chapter will be devoted to answering, in light of current knowledge, those questions most frequently asked by anesthesiologists who are approaching a hypertensive.

What are the minimal preoperative physical examination and laboratory requirements for a patient with essential hypertension?

In order to adequately assess the risk for any single patient, that patient must be categorized into a class, and conclusions and predictions drawn from epidemiologic data of that class. History is of paramount importance. Questions should be asked about exertional dyspnea, angina, overt congestive heart failure, and epistaxis. A history of stroke is important in planning the anesthetic, since, as will be amplified later, neurologic invalidism appears to be a contraindication to lowering the hypertensive's blood pressure during the course of anesthesia. Physical examination should take in all evidence of atherosclerosis. The eyegrounds are an ideal reflection of the state of this pathologic process. If the anesthesiologist does not feel confident with this examination (and many are not), a qualified internist or ophthalmologist should evaluate the patient.

A recent ECG is mandatory. Primary concern should be directed towards evidence of left ventricular hypertrophy. Manifestations of atherosclerosis, such as conduction defects and myocardial infarction, should be ruled out. A chest film provides information relevant to pulmonary infiltrates caused by congestive heart failure and also gives a direct reading of heart size.

Pertinent laboratory studies are essential to providing information to calculate overall risk. The degree of renal involvement can be demonstrated by a plasma creatinine (preferably a creatinine clearance) and urine protein. Blood urea nitrogen (BUN), although of benefit, is not as accurate for assessment as a creatinine. Plasma sodium and chloride should be obtained, but are not as mandatory as a determination of plasma potassium.

What are the criteria for proceeding with surgery in the hypertensive? When should the operative procedure be delayed?

The object of therapy is to control the hypertension. If the anesthesiologist, in his preoperative rounds, encounters an adequately controlled hypertensive without the complications of atherosclerosis, minimal physical and laboratory work should be performed, and the surgery and anesthesia should be carried out. In fact, this represents the ideal circumstance. Unfortunately, this utopian state is not always encountered.

If there is suspicion that the hypertension is not adequately treated, or that more thorough evaluation of the patient is required, the surgical procedure should be delayed, pending acquisition of data. A knowledgeable internist should be consulted. He is specifically charged with determining when the individual hypertensive is in optimal condition for surgery. He is not responsible for dictating the type of anesthesia or surgical technique: these aspects of patient care are the responsibility of the anesthesiologist and surgeon. Only when the internist believes the patient's disease is as controlled as can be, should surgery proceed. Even in these times of fiscal austerity, good medical practice demands delay while the resolution of the disease state is awaited. Obviously, there are gray zones relating to the patient who is not quite adequately treated, and resolution of such problems falls into the area of safe clinical judgment.

Emergency surgery in the untreated or inadequately treated hypertensive falls into a different category. Surgery for life-threatening conditions cannot be delayed. Under these conditions, safe anesthetic management is more difficult and will be described later.

What about antihypertensive medications? Should they be continued or stopped prior to anesthesia?

Table 1 summarizes popular antihypertensives, mechanisms of action, and side effects. The general rule is that necessary antihypertensive medications should be continued up until the time of anesthesia. Several years ago it was in vogue to withdraw such drugs several weeks prior to the surgical event. In light of present evidence, this is fallacious. The cardinal rule is that the treated, adequately controlled hypertensive is the ideal. Withdrawing antihypertensives makes as much sense as withholding all insulin from a diabetic 2 weeks before surgery. However, it is incumbent upon the anesthesiologist that he or she be cognizant of the special pharmacologic alterations produced by antihypertensive medications. Table 1 is a guide, but it is not a substitute for in-depth knowledge of common drugs used in therapy of essential hypertension.

A special note of caution should be given concerning the drug clonidine (Catapres). Abrupt withdrawal (i.e., in 8 to 24 hours) can produce a severe, life-threatening hypertensive crisis. If a patient is currently taking clonidine, the first consideration is to assess the type of surgical procedure. If it is one in which the probability that the patient will be able to take oral medications soon after surgery is high, the clonidine should be given with a

Table 1. Antihypertensive Medications in Current Use.

Drug	Mechanism of Action	Side Effects
Propranolol (Inderal)	Reduction in cardiac output.Desensitization of baroreceptors. Inhibition of renin-aldosterone system.	Resistant bradycardia. Negative inotropic action. AV conduction defects.Asthma.
Thiazide diuretics	Direct vasodepressor effects on vascular smooth muscle. Possible depletion of extracellular fluid.	Hyperglycemia. Hypokalemia. Volume depletion.
Guanethidine (Ismelin)	Depletion of post-ganglionic adrenergic nerve norepinephrine content (reserpine-like action). Inhibition of norepinephrine release by adrenergic nerves (bretylium-like effect).	Blunting of sympathetic homeostatic reflexes. Increased capacitance volume. Blunting of indirectly acting sympathetic amines (e.g., ephedrine).
Methyldopa (Aldomet)	Central nervous system vasomotor depressant action. Possible production of peripheral "false transmitter." Preservation of renal blood flow.	Sedation. Bradycardia. Reduction in MAC. Possible liver injury in certain patients.
Clonidine (Catapres)	Central inhibition of sympathetic nervous system. Preservation of renal blood flow.	Sedation. Hypertensive crisis, frequently severe or abrupt withdrawal.
Hydralazine (Apresoline)	Direct depression of vascular smooth muscle.	Tachycardia with increase in angina. Good parenteral antihypertensive effect.

small amount of water an hour or so prior to induction of anesthesia and continued postoperatively. On the other hand, if gastrointestinal surgery or other procedures in which the likelihood the patient will remain unable to take anything by mouth is contemplated, preoperative transition to parenteral antihypertensives is mandatory. Such transition will delay surgery and obviously falls within the scope of the internist.

Another drug of controversy is the beta-adrenergic receptor blocker, propranolol. In the past, there were fears expressed that this drug would produce recalcitrant hypotension during anesthesia. Prys-Roberts has performed human experiments in which he has demonstrated rather conclusively that hypertensive patients receiving beta-adrenergic receptor blockade tolerate anesthesia well. The current consensus is that propranolol should not be withdrawn. Providing the patient is adequately atropinized (heart rate is greater than 60/min), anesthesia can be safely performed in these individuals. Obviously, great care should be exercised during anesthetic management. In the author's opinion, a nitrous oxide-relaxant-thiopental-narcotic sequence with the addition of increments of halogenated anesthetics (i.e., "titration") is an extremely useful technique for this group.

The one exception to the rule of continuing medications is the monoamine oxidase (MAO) inhibitors. The use of MAO inhibitors in therapy of hypertension is unusual these days, and few patients using them are seen. The best available advice is to discontinue MAO inhibitors 2 weeks prior to surgery and provide transition to another antihypertensive regimen. If surgery is emergent in a patient on this class of drugs, a nitrous oxide-thiopental-relaxant sequence is probably best. Meperidine (Demerol) and indirectly acting sympathetic amines (ephedrine) must be assiduously avoided since they may precipitate a severe hypertensive crisis.

Where should I keep the blood pressure during anesthesia? What are the best anesthetic techniques?

These are obviously pragmatic and thought-provoking questions, which are not completely answerable with current information. The role of regional anesthesia has not been definitely established. Certainly, peripheral nerve blocks are indicated.

The high spinal or peridural block intrinsically possesses far less blood pressure controllability than does "titration" with a volatile inhalation anesthetic. Clinical judgment and experience play a great role in determining the technique of greatest safety for the particular patient.

The author prefers the use of potent inhalation anesthetics, such as halothane and enflurane, since blood pressures, except for certain circumstances discussed later, are best held at near control levels. High blood pressures are dangerous and should be carefully avoided. Addition of small increments of potent anesthetics in order to judge responses are favored. In patients with hypertensive renal disease, it may be prudent to avoid enflurane and methoxyflurane. Hypokalemia should be corrected preoperatively, since it may provoke serious disturbances of cardiac rhythm and may enhance neuromuscular blockade. Metabolic alkalosis from potassium depletion also depresses ventilation postoperatively. In the adequately treated hypertensive, intraoperative blood pressures should be maintained close to preoperative values.

The untreated hypertensive patient who requires emergency surgery represents a special category when determining the best level at which to maintain blood pressure. Unfortunately, precise data concerning optimum levels of blood pressure in these circumstances are lacking. Certain extrapolations from nonanesthetized hypertensives probably represent correct assumptions, however. High blood pressure is destructive. Elevated levels of peripheral resistance cause increased afterload on the myocardium and predispose to congestive heart failure. Likewise, stroke is facilitated by hypertension. Nonanesthetized patients in hypertensive crisis are benefited by abrupt reductions in blood pressure. Myocardial work is decreased, myocardial oxygenation is improved, and cerebrovascular spasm is decreased. Perhaps the organ most sensitive to rapid decreases in blood pressure is the kidney. Autoregulation in the kidney does not appear to be as rapid as that in the brain and heart. An underlying arteriolar nephrosclerosis may be unmasked by precipitous declines in blood pressure. However, overall, it would seem prudent to decrease the diastolic blood pressure to within 20 percent of "normal" levels in most cases of untreated hypertensives who are scheduled for emergency surgery. This can usually be done with an anesthetic such as halothane. About the only circumstance in which this might be contraindicated is in the patient with neurologic disease secondary to hypertension and/or atherosclerosis. These individuals may not have sufficient reserve cerebral autoregulation and are quite dependent upon pressure for perfusion.

A word or two should be mentioned concerning administration of fluid during surgical procedures in the hypertensive. One of the salient features of potent inhalation anesthetics is reduction in peripheral resistance, accompanied by an increased capacitance volume. Since sympathetic compensatory reflexes are obtunded by these anesthetics, volume becomes of extreme importance insofar as blood pressure is concerned. Two features of the hypertensive patient are of importance in this regard. First, unless there is concomitant renal dysfunction, the essential hypertensive patient can handle a sodium load as well as the normotensive patient. Second, many treated and untreated hypertensives may have diminished blood volumes and/or extracellular fluid volumes. The conclusion to be drawn from these data is that judicious use of salt-containing solutions, such as Ringer's lactate, may be of great value in maintaining blood pressure and organ perfusion. The use of volume rather than sympathomimetic amines to prevent serious hypotension is to be recommended.

What is the drug of choice to combat hypertension in the recovery room?

The assumption is made that the patient is one with a diagnosis of hypertension, who has a marked rise in blood pressure following surgery and elimination of vasodepressant drugs, such as volatile anesthetics. Obviously, a certain diagnostic acumen is necessary in this condition. Causes of hypertension in the recovery room include hypoxia, hypercapnia, urinary retention, and pain. Rebound drug withdrawal (i.e., clonidine) is handled quite differently and must be excluded. These precipitating factors must be ruled out. If the blood pressure elevation is clearly due to essential hypertension rebound, there are several therapeutic possibilities. In the absence of angina, the author's favorite drug is hydralazine, administered in 2.5 to 5.0 mg increments intravenously. A waiting period of 10 to 15 minutes should be allowed between incremental doses. Usually no more than 20 mg will be required. Nitroprusside infusion may be employed, but this necessitates intra-arterial monitoring, and the patient requires much closer observation in the recovery room than when hydralazine is employed.

BIBLIOGRAPHY

Crout, J. R., and Brown, B. R., Jr.: *Anesthesia and the hypertensive patient.* Clin. Anesthesiol. 3:152, 1969.

Freis, E. D.: *The clinical spectrum of hypertension.* Arch. Int. Med. 133:982-987, 1974

Holland, O. B., and Kaplan, N. M.: *Propranolol in treatment of hypertension.* N. Engl. J. Med. 294:930, 1976.

Prys-Roberts, C., Foex, P., Biro, G. P., et al.: *Studies of anesthetic in relation to hypertension. V. Adrenergic beta receptor blockade.* Br. J. Anaesth. 45:671, 680, 1973.

Tarazi, R. C., Frohlich, E. D., and Dustan, H. P.: *Plasma volume in men with essential hypertension.* N. Engl. J. Med. 278:762, 1968.

Veterans Administration Study on Antihypertensive Agents: *Effects of treatment on morbidity in hypertension.* J.A.M.A. 202:1028, 1967.

HYPOTENSION DURING NONCARDIAC ANESTHESIA IN THE CARDIAC PATIENT

G. Y. Gaines, M.D., and
A. H. Giesecke, M.D.

Drs. Gaines and Giesecke present a major portion of the diorama of hypotensive occurrences during anesthesia in the cardiac patient. Both diagnosis and current therapy of each type of episode are discussed by them.

Burnell R. Brown, Jr.

Heart disease is widely known to be the number one cause of morbidity and mortality in the United States. This statement refers primarily to coronary artery disease, although it also includes hypertension, valvular disease, and other cardiac abnormalities.[1] The risk of anesthesia and surgery is greater in patients with coronary disease than in other forms of heart disease. The mortality increases with advancing age, length of surgical procedure, and extent of the surgical procedure.[2] A collected series by Nachlas and coworkers[3] revealed a mortality rate of 2.9 percent in noncardiac patients and a mortality rate of 6.6 percent in cardiac patients. These figures represent more than a twofold increase in mortality in patients with organic heart disease.

The perioperative morbidity and mortality of patients with coronary artery disease who are undergoing noncardiac surgery are said to have improved since the dawn of coronary artery surgery. Surgeons and anesthetists have gained an enormous amount of experience in caring for patients with coronary artery disease. The validity of such a statement requires objective substantiation, and at the moment the assumption appears extremely tenuous. As recently as 1975, Sapala, Ponka, and Duvernoy[4] reported an 83 percent mortality rate (six of seven patients) when the electrocardiographic interpretation was consistent with recent acute myocardial infarction. A major reason for the low mortality figures with coronary artery operations *may be* that myocardial revascularization immediately improves blood supply and oxygen supply to heart muscle. Such is not the case when a gallbladder is removed or a hip is replaced.

Before we can consider the causes, prevention, sequelae, or treatment of hypotension, we must define the term in the context in which it is employed in clinical practice. Normotension is defined as normal tension or normal blood pressure. Based on statistical data gathered from observation on apparently "normal, healthy" young patients, the acceptable expected blood pressure is approximately 120/80 torr, with the normal heart rate being approximately 72 beats per minute. Apparently, blood pressure readings and heart rates in this range must be most beneficial because vital end-organ perfusion is accomplished without undue demand on the myocardium. Significant deviation from these ranges of blood pressure and heart rate have never been shown to be beneficial and have frequently been illustrated to be detrimental.

Hypotension may be defined as diminished tension or lowered blood pressure. Blood pressure significantly lower than the normal range may be assumed to subject the individual to the hazards of decreased perfusion of vital end-organs. Atherosclerosis of the vascular bed of various vital organs, such as the heart and brain, interferes with autoregulation and causes flow to become more dependent on blood pressure. Myocardial infarction and cerebral vascular accidents are expected sequelae of significant falls in blood pressure.

Hypertension is defined as elevated tension or elevated blood pressure. The unfortunate sequelae of long-term hypertension are very well known to the medical community, and the lay population as well. Until very recently, however, the assumption was made that short periods of hypertension and tachycardia in the patient suffering from cardiac disease or vascular disease were not detrimental and may actually be beneficial to the maintenance of end-organ blood flow. Information gained from fairly recent laboratory and clinical studies has shown that, especially in a patient population afflicted with coronary artery disease, intrinsic myocardial disease, or generalized atherosclerosis, one must attempt to maintain adequate organ perfusion and oxygen supply without unduly increasing myocardial oxygen consumption.

MYOCARDIAL OXYGEN CONSUMPTION

Briefly, the major determinants of myocardial oxygen consumption are as follows[5]:

1. *External work* is the product of mean arterial blood pressure (often termed afterload) and cardiac output. The heart requires more oxygen to perform pressure work than volume work. Oxygen consumption doubles when pressure work doubles, but increases only 25 percent when cardiac output doubles. Therefore, simply stated, as blood pressure increases, myocardial oxygen consumption increases.
2. *Internal work* is developed chamber tension or the product of pressure and radius, based on Laplace's law, which relates intraluminal tension to chamber size.

3. *Heart rate,* when increased, will reduce diastolic time. At rest, 70 percent of the coronary flow occurs during diastole. As heart rate increases, myocardial oxygen consumption increases at a time when coronary flow may be decreasing.
4. *Contractile state* is perhaps best expressed as intrinsic ventricular compliance. It can be defined as that property of heart muscle that characterizes the force of contraction independent of preload or afterload. That is, for any level of contractile state, the extent of fiber shortening will vary directly with the preload and inversely with the afterload.
5. *Basal metabolic rate* refers to the relatively insignificant amount of oxygen that is consumed during diastole.
6. *Electrical activity* requires very small amounts of oxygen, but for completeness' sake this amount must be included.

Now we must consider the factors determining the availability of oxygen to the myocardium. They are as follows:

1. Oxygen content of arterial blood
2. Coronary blood flow, which, in turn, is determined by:
   a. Perfusion pressure
   b. Autoregulation
   c. Effective blood viscosity

Basically, availability of oxygen to the myocardium may be expressed as the product of coronary blood flow and arterial oxygen content.

Increased metabolic demand in most body tissues can be met by increasing oxygen extraction, which is evidenced by widening of the arteriovenous oxygen difference. This is not true with the myocardium. Virtually all the oxygen is extracted from the arterial blood under resting conditions. The implication of this fact is that any increase in myocardial work must be met by a commensurate increase in coronary blood flow.

Regional distribution is of critical importance. Blood flow to the subendocardium may be severely compromised despite an adequate total coronary flow. The amount of blood delivered to any area of the myocardium is determined by the difference between intraluminal and extraluminal pressures, that is, the driving force minus the intramural wall tension.

Resistance to flow is regulated by vasomotor tone and modified by shearing forces, blood viscosity, and right atrial pressure (offering obstruction to coronary sinus drainage). In diseased vessels, however, the picture is complicated by the fact that flow is no longer luminal and many of the physical laws do not apply. Where localized narrowing is present in the coronary vessels, flow to the distal (i.e., potentially ischemic) areas is highly pressure-dependent. When vessels in the area of a perfusion deficit dilate in response to local metabolic activity, the velocity of flow distal to the obstruction is reduced. Thus, a fall in driving pressure may result in a marked degree of stasis in the microcirculation.

Studies have shown that the majority of myocardial oxygen consumption is related to the product of heart rate and peak systolic blood pressure (the rate-pressure product.) In the clinical situation, myocardial oxygen consumption is elevated when heart rate is increased or when peak systolic pressure is raised owing to an increase in peripheral resistance with either elevated or unchanged cardiac output. An increase in cardiac output may be attained without an increase in oxygen consumption, if peak systolic pressure is lowered and heart rate is not proportionately increased.[6]

The rate-pressure product furnishes an important clinical guide for the anesthesiologist. The vast majority of patients with significant myocardial disease of any variety, but especially coronary artery disease, will develop anginal chest pain or ischemic changes on the V-leads of the electrocardiogram when the rate-pressure product is allowed to exceed the 12,000 to 15,000 range.[7] The anesthesiologist must maintain his patient's blood pressure and heart rate as near the normal range as possible in order to sustain adequate organ perfusion on one hand and avoid unwarranted increase in myocardial oxygen consumption on the other.

As one approaches a specific discussion of hypotension during noncardiac anesthesia in the cardiac patient, the realization emerges that the causes of hypotension in this patient population are not different from those acting in patients who are free of known cardiac disease. However, while the etiologies of hypotension in the perianesthetic period may be similar in all patients, the cardiac patient is more likely to experience hypotension and much more likely to suffer untoward sequelae as a result of hypotension than is the patient without cardiac problems. Simply stated, because of disease processes affecting the cardiovascular system or the presence of therapeutic medications, the patient suffering from heart disease may not be capable of compensating for hypotension in a healthy manner by increasing cardiac output and/or peripheral vascular resistance.

In order to intelligently approach the differential diagnosis of hypotension occurring in conjunction with any type of anesthetic administration, one must have available a classification that is easy to recall. Although we are discussing hypotension and not shock, Shires's[8] modification of the classification of shock offered by Blalock in 1934[9] serves very well as a foundation for this approach. The perianesthetic period presents many stresses that may be considered as contributing factors to the development of hypotension. These contributing factors will correspond to the major categories in Blalock's classification.

For clinical purposes three etiologic categories of hypotension may be developed:

1. *Cardiogenic hypotension* refers to that which results from a fall in cardiac output. The following factors may contribute to a decline in cardiac output:
   a. Preanesthetic medications
   b. Therapeutic medications
   c. General anesthetic agents and adjuncts
   d. Local anesthetic agents
   e. Cardiac catastrophies
   f. Surgical manipulations
2. *Hypovolemic hypotension* refers to a decline in blood pressure secondary to a lack of effective volume for the heart to pump. Contributing factors are:
   a. Blood loss
   b. Plasma loss
   c. Water and electrolyte loss
3. *Vasogenic hypotension* denotes decreased vascular tone, on both arterial and venous sides of the circulation, as the source of hypotension. The diminished vascular tone may result from direct effects on the smooth muscle in the vessel wall or from neurogenic influences on the vascular smooth muscle. Factors tending to affect vascular tone in the circumstances of anesthetic administration are many:
   a. Preanesthetic medications
   b. Therapeutic medications

c. General anesthetic agents and adjuncts
d. Local anesthetic agents
e. Spinal and peridural anesthesia
f. Vascular accidents
g. Surgical manipulations
h. Elevated airway pressure
i. Patient position
j. Sepsis
k. Anaphylaxis
l. Hemolytic transfusion reaction

Hypotension may occur secondary to a multitude of etiologies, all coming into play in varying degrees, simultaneously. Now that we have a working clinical guideline for the differential diagnosis of hypotension in conjunction with the perianesthetic period, it is appropriate to discuss in some detail the specific etiologic factors as they relate to the patient suffering from cardiac disease.

SPECIFIC ETIOLOGIC FACTORS

Premedication

Proper premedication is no simple task in the cardiac patient. Catecholamine release, which may result from undue apprehension, may produce elevation of heart rate and blood pressure sufficient to provoke angina or myocardial infarction. On the other hand, overly heavy premedication with the opiates may lower arterial pressure by several pharmacologic actions: depression of the vasomotor center, reduction in skeletal muscle tone, and dilation of peripheral blood vessels owing to a direct action or secondary to release of histamine. The barbiturates, in excessive doses, may markedly lower blood pressure secondary to myocardial or vascular depression.

The premedication regimen employed at our institution consists of an unhurried, frank, and detailed discussion of the planned anesthetic management followed by diazepam 0.1 to 0.2 mg/kg by mouth and morphine 0.1 to 0.2 mg/kg intramuscularly 45 minutes before the patient is to arrive in the operating room. If desired, scopolamine 0.4 mg intramuscularly may be added for its amnesic effect and for its tendency to slow the heart rate. The specific premedication plan must be tailored to fit the particular patient, but our experience has demonstrated lack of significant respiratory or cardiovascular depression associated with this combination of drugs.

Therapeutic Drugs Employed Prior to Anesthesia

Some drugs employed in modern therapeutics can affect the course of anesthesia unfavorably, as regards cardiovascular instability. This is particularly true of medications that may be administered to the cardiac patient.

The antihypertensive drugs may potentiate the reduction in blood pressure often noted with general anesthetics. The mechanism may be depletion of norepinephrine at the sympathetic postganglionic nerve terminal or at the vascular smooth muscle cell (guanethidine), or a direct relaxing effect on the vascular smooth muscle in the wall of the vessels (hydralazine).

The beta-adrenergic blockers (generally propranolol) employed in the treatment of angina, hypertension, and cardiac dysrhythmias may markedly decrease myocardial contractility, especially when they are in the company of anesthetic agents that are capable of myocardial depression.

Finally, many tranquilizers, administered to cardiac patients to allay anxiety, are capable of disturbing catecholamine metabolism and thus promoting cardiovascular instability. Even diuretic agents employed in treatment of hypertension or congestive heart failure may reduce effective volume of extracellular fluid to a degree that may cause the patient to become very susceptible to any potential cause of hypotension.[10]

For many years, the recommendation was made that these drugs should be withheld for several days, or even weeks, prior to anesthesia and surgery in order to avoid their hypotensive effects. Recent studies and clinical experience indicate that withdrawal of these necessary therapeutic medications may provoke an exacerbation of the basic cardiovascular disease process just as the patient is about to face the physiologic ordeal of anesthesia and surgery.[11]

Current accepted practice tends to continue most therapeutic agents necessary to control the disease state up until 4 to 6 hours prior to anesthesia, while it keeps in mind the potential untoward effects of these agents and is prepared to treat them, should they arise, with fluid and pharmacologic support of the cardiovascular system.

General Anesthetics

Administration of general inhalation anesthetic agents is a common cause of fall in arterial blood pressure, especially in patients suffering from heart disease. The drop in blood pressure may be the result of a relative rather than an absolute overdose. The pharmacologic response to progressive deepening of anesthesia with all currently employed general anesthetics entails peripheral vasodilatation and reduced myocardial contractility.[12]

Nitrous oxide, long thought of as a benign agent demonstrating some slight sympathetic response and little change in hemodynamics in normal patients, has been shown to cause quite severe myocardial depression in patients with heart disease.[13]

Many of the commonly employed intravenous drugs used to induce, maintain, or supplement general anesthesia are very capable of producing hypotension. The thiobarbiturates are well known for their ability to depress the cardiovascular system[14]; d-tubocurarine produces peripheral vascular dilatation by way of ganglionic blockade and histamine release.[15]

Even ketamine, famous for the increased heart rate, blood pressure, systemic vascular resistance, and myocardial contractility it causes, may exert a direct myocardial depressant effect in the presence of complete beta-receptor blockade.[16]

Arterial hypotension in the presence of general anesthetic agents or adjuncts may be prevented by administering the least amount of anesthetic compatible with adequate surgical conditions, taking the time to induce anesthesia gradually or to change from one level to another slowly, and judiciously using fluids or drugs to support the cardiovascular system.

Local Anesthetic Agents

Very frequently some form of local infiltration, nerve block, or topical anesthesia is recommended for the patient with cardiac disease. This is done to avoid the systemic effects of a general anesthetic; however, inadvertant absorption of local anesthetic agents from mucous membranes or other highly vascular tissues may cause marked hypotension. Probable causes of lowered blood pressure include depression of the myocardium and the vasomotor centers, as well as dilation of peripheral vessels as a result of direct action.[17] Although prior administration of a barbiturate does not protect against these effects, diazepam premedication in cats increases the dose of local anesthetic tolerated prior to convulsion.

Hypotension can be minimized by reducing the total quantity of anesthetic injected per unit of time. Use of large volumes of concentrated solutions and rapid injection are chiefly responsible for dangerous elevation of blood levels. When topical anesthesia is used, the same principles apply. Application is performed slowly to avoid rapid vascular absorption.

Should significant fall in blood pressure occur, treatment involves oxygen supplementation of inspired gases and intravenous fluid and pharmacologic support of the cardiovascular system.

Spinal and Peridural Anesthesia

The mechanisms for the fall in blood pressure often observed after spinal and peridural anesthesia are a reduction in total peripheral resistance, which results from paralysis of sympathetic vasoconstrictor fibers to arterioles and venules, and a decline in cardiac output in response to a reduction of venous return to the heart consequent to pooling of blood in the dilated capacitance vessels.[18] A precipitous fall in blood pressure may occur after spinal or peridural anesthesia in the patient with cardiac disease because of reduced extracellular fluid volume, diminished vascular reactivity, and decreased ability to effectively increase cardiac output. In order to prevent a catastrophe that may be associated with a sudden reduction of blood pressure in this high risk patient population, the anesthetist must recognize that hypotension can develop immediately upon intrathecal injection of the local anesthetic solution. Treatment must be prompt!

Intravenous fluid therapy and vasopressor agents are the cornerstones of treatment for hypotension associated with spinal and peridural anesthesia. However, in this fragile group, overzealous use of intravenous fluids may easily lead to congestive heart failure; heavy-handed use of vasopressor agents may sharply increase myocardial oxygen consumption as a result of a positive inotropic effect or undue increase in peripheral resistance. The intelligent management of this problem requires a multifaceted approach.

First, spinal or peridural anesthesia must be determined to be appropriate for the extent of the surgical field. If the surgical field dictates a sensory dermatomic blockade to the upper thoracic segments, the accompanying sympathetic blockade would be expected to produce a striking degree of cardiovascular instability. Another anesthetic technique might be more appropriate in this instance.

Second, intravenous fluids, such as 200 to 500 ml of lactated Ringer's solution, may be employed to bolster effective extracellular fluid volume to ward off or attenuate hypotension.[19] However, this form of treatment might be unwarranted in the circumstances of impending congestive heart failure or decreased renal function. In these circumstances, elevation of the patient's legs will promote venous drainage to the right heart. The entire body should not be tilted head down, lest a higher level of anesthesia develop.

Finally, the third and possibly most rational therapy for this patient group is appropriate use of vasopressor agents. Intravenous administration combined with low incremental dosage allows the benefit of rapid onset of action without the danger of sustained iatrogenic hypertension. Since the altered physiology is primarily one of decreased peripheral resistance, a pure alpha-adrenergic agent, such as methoxamine or phenylephrine, would seem indicated. At our institution, 10 mg phenylephrine in 500 ml of D5W, administered by microdrip, and methoxamine diluted to 2 mg per ml, administered incrementally I.V. have proven very effective. Should the heart rate slow below 70 beats per minute, glycopyrrolate administered in 0.1-mg increments intravenously may effectively support heart rate without provoking a sustained tachycardia.

Spinal or peridural anesthesia may have much to offer the patient with heart disease, but this is true only if hypotension is prevented or appropriately treated.

Cardiovascular Catastrophies

In a patient with cardiac disease, some type of cardiovascular catastrophe would be a likely cause of severe hypotension. Bradycardia, tachycardia, dysrhythmias, ischemia, infarction, acute congestive failure, valvular incompetency, cardiac tamponade, and rupture of a ventricular aneurysm would all result in hypotension under anesthesia.

Embolism to any of several vascular beds may lead to hypotension, the cause of which may not be easily determined. Cerebral embolism, pulmonary embolism from peripheral veins, fat embolism from fracture sites, amniotic fluid emboli during delivery, and venous air embolism during upright cervical operations or craniotomy may all provoke severe cardiovascular instability.

Onset of any form of cardiovascular decompensation in these fragile patients constitutes the gravest medical emergency and demands, in most cases, prompt, heroic supportive treatment if the patient is to survive.

Hypovolemia

Arterial hypotension is the logical sequela of loss of blood, plasma, or fluid and electrolytes from the dynamics of circulation, whatever the cause. In this patient population, meticulous maintenance of intraoperative fluid balance is an absolute necessity in order to tread the thin line between hypotension and congestive heart failure. Compulsive measurement of intraoperative blood loss and constant monitoring of pulse rate, arterial pressure, central venous pressure, urine output, and possibly pulmonary artery pressure are all essential if the anesthetist is to provide proper fluid balance.

One must always remember that the cardiovascular depressant effects of many anesthetic agents may combine with only moderate hypovolemia to produce striking degrees of hypotension. Careful control of anesthetic administration, constant monitoring of parameters reflecting fluid volume and cardiovascular function, and conservative intravenous fluid therapy are the principles most likely to produce a beneficial result as far as intraoperative fluid balance is concerned.

Elevated Airway Pressure

Positive pressure applied to the airway may lower arterial pressure. Raised airway pressure is transmitted to the large intrathoracic blood vessels and to the pulmonary capillaries as well. The higher the mean pressure, the lower the blood flow through these vessels, and cardiac output diminishes in proportion to the degree of interference with venous return. As cardiac output and arterial pressure fall, compensatory vasoconstriction in

both venous and arterial circulations is initiated via baroreceptor discharge.[20] A normal individual can tolerate reasonable degrees of raised airway pressure through this ability to constrict
peripheral vessels, especially those of the venous capacitance
system.

This phenomenon is very significant in the patient with cardiac disease who is subjected to general anesthesia. The cardiovascular response to raised airway pressure in this patient population may be potentiated by cardiovascular depressant effects of anesthetic agents, hypovolemia secondary to diuretic
therapy, antihypertensive medications that interfere with appropriate increases in peripheral vascular resistance, and beta-
blocker therapy and/or myocardial disease, which limit appropriate compensatory changes in cardiac output.

Basic treatment of this problem consists of decreasing the
level and duration of pressure applied to the airway. During the
period of general anesthetic administration, gentle manual ventilation may be substituted for mechanical ventilation.

Surgical Maneuvers

Surgical manipulation in the neck, thorax, or abdomen is a common cause of arterial hypotension, which may be explained on
a mechanical or reflex basis. The fall in blood pressure is more
likely to occur and more likely to be significant in the environment of a diseased cardiovascular system.

Hypotension may reflexively follow traction on the gallbladder, bowel, uterus, or mesentery; or stimulation of the perito-
neum, periosteum, joint cavities, carotid sinus, or various struc-
tures in the chest. The autonomic nervous system is presumed
to be involved in these reactions, but the exact neural pathways
are often not clear. However, as a result of afferent impulses,
both inhibition of sympathetic activity and increased vagal tone
on the heart have been shown. Atrial contraction contributes to
ventricular filling, and vagal-induced reduction in contractility
may participate in the diminished stroke volume observed. A
puzzling aspect of the hypotension observed during surgical activity is the absence of bradycardia on some occasions and its
presence at other times. Peripheral vasodilatation may play a
role in some instances.

Venous return to the heart may be obstructed by surgical

packs, clamps, torsion or compression of large veins by retractors, gallbladder or kidney rests, or by pressure of the gravid uterus or large abdominal tumors upon the inferior vena cava. Rapid release of increased intra-abdominal pressure during drainage of ascites or delivery of a large abdominal tumor may be followed by hypotension as a result of sudden expansion of the mesenteric venous bed. Rapid decompression of a distended urinary bladder may cause hypotension by this mechanism.

Finally, serious hypotension may result when a surgeon removes clamps from the aorta or applies a large volume of poorly cured methyl methacrylate cement to a bone marrow cavity.

Gentleness on the part of surgeons and awareness by all concerned of the consequences of their maneuvers constitute the basis for prevention and treatment of hypotension resulting from surgical manipulation. The anesthetist must be aware of surgical action at all times and be prepared to instantly inform the surgical team of any untoward physiologic response on the part of the patient.

Patient Position

The circulation of the anesthetized patient is less able to compensate for stress than that of the unanesthetized one, particularly in those patients with severe cardiovascular disease.

The assumption of any position that promotes gravitational pooling of blood in the peripheral vascular bed may be expected to produce a fall in arterial pressure; the mechanism is decreased venous return to the right heart with fall in cardiac output. This phenomenon would be especially likely to occur with assumption of the lateral decubitus with flexion and the sitting positions.

Prevention consists of slow, gentle positioning, wrapping of the legs with Ace bandages, and applying careful fluid and pharmacologic support to the cardiovascular system.[21]

Hemolytic Transfusion Reaction

In the perianesthetic period, unexplained hypotension and oozing from the surgical site, accompanying administration of red cells, must strongly suggest incompatible transfusion until proven otherwise. Initial treatment, at least, consists of discontinuing the transfusion and checking the plasma and urine for free hemoglobin.

Septic Shock

Septic shock rarely appears for the first time during anesthesia and operation. Either it is present preoperatively and operation is attempted in the hope of removing the source of infection, or it develops postoperatively owing to spread of a previously contained infection or contamination of a wound.

A detailed discussion of the treatment of septic shock is beyond the scope of this article, but involves standard supportive therapy, control of fever, antibiotics, vasodilator agents, fluid therapy, massive corticosteroid therapy, and cardiotonic agents, such as digitalis, isoproterenol, or dopamine.[22] The acute onset of septic shock during surgery and anesthesia in a patient with cardiac disease would spell a very grim prognosis, indeed.

Anaphylactic Reaction

This phenomenon is a very uncommon cause of hypotension noted by anesthetists. Some degree of protection against anaphylaxis, afforded by general anesthetics, has been demonstrated, but the protection is only against the more mild degree of reaction.

Anaphylaxis is one form of immediate allergic response involving circulating antibodies in the serum of a patient and extrinsic antigens. Treatment consists of the administration of oxygen, epinephrine parenterally, bronchodilators, and steroids. Antihistamines tend to be of limited value, and then only if administered very early in the reaction.[23]

MANAGEMENT OF HYPOTENSION

We have discussed in some detail the etiologies and appropriate treatment of hypotension when it occurs in the cardiac patient during the perianesthetic period. However, certain broad principles must be applied to the treatment of hypotension in these circumstances, if our patients are to survive to undergo more sophisticated management.

First, meticulous, detailed preoperative preparation is an absolute necessity in this patient population. Pulmonary function, fluid balance, electrolytic status, and all therapeutic manipulation should be tuned to an optimal degree; only in this manner may the cardiac patient's limited physiologic and anatomic reserves be at a maximum level as he faces the ordeal of anesthesia and surgery.

Next, monitoring of as many parameters as possible that are related to the state of the cardiovascular system should be applied to these patients. Measurement of arterial blood pressure, pulse, central venous pressure, pulmonary artery pressure, urinary output, and arterial blood gas values may yield information of aid to the anesthesiologist; this information may warn of impending hypotension, point to a particular etiology, or allow rapid evaluation of the results of a particular form of treatment.

Finally, if hypotension does occur in this patient population, no matter the anesthetic method employed, prompt, heroic measures must be taken in order to maintain blood flow and oxygen supply to the diseased myocardium. Initial measures should be along the following lines:

Oxygen Therapy

Maximum levels of inspired oxygen should be administered while diagnosis and therapy are being performed. If general anesthetic agents are being administered, they should be markedly reduced in concentration or completely discontinued. If some form of conduction anesthetic is being employed, manual ventilation by way of mask or quickly placed endotracheal tube may be necessary.

Intravenous Fluids

Rapid intravenous administration of blood or other fluids may, of course, be appropriate during severe hypotension. However, in the cardiac patient, vigorous administration of fluid should be reserved for treating hypotension secondary to acute hemorrhage or loss of extracellular fluid. Injudicious use of intravenous fluids in this clinical setting may lead to further deterioration of myocardial function and worsening of hypotension.

Vasopressors

Careful application of vasopressor therapy early in the episode of hypotension may be very appropriate in this patient population. Many drugs are available, but they should be employed according to their specific mechanism of action.

As noted previously in this discussion, if hypotension exists primarily because of vasodilation, as following spinal or peridural anesthesia, a pressor agent such as neosynephrine or methoxamine, both with an action primarily on peripheral blood vessels, should be considered the drug of choice.

Should hypotension develop during the administration of an inhalation anesthetic, an agent capable of increasing myocardial contractility may be appropriate. Ephedrine 5 to 10 mg intravenously; isoproterenol 0.4 to 0.8 mg in 500 cc dextrose in water administered by microdrip; or dopamine 200 mg in 500 cc dextrose in water administered by microdrip have all been employed with advantage in the treatment of hypotension. Dopamine offers some potential advantage in low dose, as it may increase myocardial contractility without producing renal vasoconstriction.[24]

Definitive Diagnosis and Treatment

Appropriate diagnosis and treatment of the etiology of hypotension should follow application of initial supportive measures.

In order to protect this fragile group of patients from the ravages of hypotension, the anesthesiologist must be knowledgeable in cardiovascular anatomy and physiology, prepare his patient optimally, monitor scrupulously, and tailor his anesthetic management appropriately. He must treat hypotension intelligently and quickly, should it occur. This is a demanding task, but one the anesthesiologist must perform, nonetheless.

REFERENCES

1. Hillis, C. D., and Braunwald, E.: *Myocardial ischemia.* N. Engl. J. Med. 296:971, 1034, and 1093, 1977.
2. Skinner, J. F., and Pearce, M. L.: *Surgical risk in the cardiac patient.* J. Chronic Dis. 17:57, 1964.

3. Nachlas, M. M., Abrams, S. J., and Goldberg, M. M.: *The influence of arteriosclerotic heart disease on surgical risk.* Am. J. Surg. 101:447, 1961.
4. Sapala, J. A., Ponka, J. L., and Duvernoy, W. F.: *Operative and non-operative risks in the cardiac patient.* J. Am. Geriatr. Soc. 23:529, 1975.
5. Braunwald, E.: *The determinants of myocardial oxygen consumption.* Physiologist 12:65, 1969.
6. Wynands, J. E., Sheridan, C. A., Batra, M. S., et al.: *Coronary artery disease.* Anesthesiology 33:260, 1970.
7. Robinson, B. F.: *Relation of heart rate and systolic blood pressure to the onset of pain and angina pectoris.* Circulation 35:1073, 1967.
8. Shires, G. T.: *Care of the Trauma Patient.* McGraw-Hill Book Co., New York, 1966, pp. 3–5.
9. Blalock, A.: *Shock, further studies with particular reference to effects of hemorrhage.* Arch. Surg. 29:837, 1934.
10. Geer, R. T.: *Anesthetic management of patients with cardiac disease.* Surg. Clin. North Am. 55:5 903, 1975.
11. Diaz, R. G., Sonnbert, J. C., Freeman, E., et al.: *Withdrawal of propranolol and myocardial infarction.* Lancet 1:1068, 1973.
12. Kenmotsu, O.: *Effect of inhalation anesthetics on myocardial contractility.* Jpn. J. Anesthesiol. 23:402, 1974.
13. Smith, N. T., Calverley, R. K., Prys-Roberts, C., et al.: *Impact of nitrous oxide on the circulation during enflurane anesthesia in man.* Anesthesiology 48:345, 1978.
14. Conway, C. M., and Ellis, D. B.: *The hemodynamic effects of short-acting barbiturates.* Br. J. Anaesth. 41:534, 1969.
15. Paton, W. D.: *The effects of muscle relaxants other than muscular relaxation.* Anesthesiology 20:453, 1959.
16. Urthaler, F., Walker, A. A., and James, T. N.: *Comparison of the inotropic action of morphine and ketamine studied in canine cardiac muscle.* J. Thorac. Cardiovasc. Surg. 72:142, 1976.
17. de Jong, R. H.: *Local Anesthetics,* ed. 2. Charles C Thomas, Springfield, Illinois, 1977, pp. 115–150.
18. Lund, P. C.: *Principles and Practice of Spinal Anesthesia,* ed. 1. Charles C Thomas, Springfield, Illinois, 1977, pp. 134–192.
19. Wollman, S. B., and Marx, G. F.: *Prevention of hypotension of spinal anesthesia in parturients by acute hydration.* Anesthesiology 29:374, 1968.
20. Scurr, C., and Feldman, S.: *Scientific Foundations of Anesthesia,* ed. 1. F. A. Davis Co., Philadelphia, 1970, p. 193.
21. Courington, F. W., and Little, D. M.: *The role of posture in anesthesia.* Clin. Anesth. 3:23, 1968.

22. Christy, J. L.: *Treatment of gram-negative shock.* Am. J. Med. 50:77, 1970.
23. Dripps, R. D., Eckenhoff, J. E., and Vandam, L. D.: *Introduction to Anesthesia—The Principles of Safe Practice,* ed. 5. W. B. Saunders Co., Philadelphia, 1977, pp. 421–422.
24. Vandam, L. D.: *"Drugs for arterial hypotension and shock."* In Modell, W. (ed.): *Drugs of Choice.* C. V. Mosby Company, St. Louis, 1976.

PREOPERATIVE EVALUATION OF PATIENTS WITH ELECTROCARDIOGRAPHIC CONDUCTION DEFECTS

Gordon A. Ewy, M.D.

Dr. Ewy, a cardiologist, explores certain arrhythmias that are of concern to the anesthesiologist. His view is somewhat different than that expressed by Dr. Atlee, an anesthesiologist. Dr. Ewy has, as his major concern, arrhythmias existing prior to anesthesia and surgery. He describes in detail newer concepts of sinus node disturbances and discusses indications for use of the artificial pacemaker.

Burnell R. Brown, Jr.

The heart is normally activated by a depolarization wave that originates in the sinoatrial (SA or sinus) node, travels the intranodal pathways, and spreads to activate the atrium. The impulse is slowed in the atrioventricular node (AV node) before rapidly traversing the bundle of His and the three fascicles of the ventricular activating system. The surface and intracardiac electrocardiographic manifestations of these electrophysiologic events are illustrated in Figure 1. Atrial depolarization is reflected in the P wave of the ECG. As the impulse travels through the AV node, the surface ECG is electrically silent (PR segment), but a small spike (H) can be recorded with an appropriately placed intracardiac catheter electrode. This impulse reflects the depolarization of the bundle of His. The QRS complex of the surface ECG and the ventricular or "V" deflections of the bipolar intracardiac recording signal the onset of ventricular activation.

The spectrum of conduction abnormalities ranges from minor slowing, to major delays, to complete block of the depolarizing impulse. These abnormalities may occur in the tissue in and around the SA node, in the AV node, and in the trifascicular conduction system. The clinical manifestations of conduction delays in these three general areas are the sick sinus syndrome, delays or block within the AV node, or block in one or more of the fascicles of the ventricular activating system.

Before reviewing these three problems and their preoperative evaluation, it is important to emphasize that conduction delays and blocks may be transient and reversible. The following are clinically important causes of conduction delays:

Physiologic

1. Increased vagal tone (SA node, atrium, and junctional tissue)
2. Decreased sympathetic tone (SA node, atrium, and junctional tissue)
3. Electrolytic abnormalities (hyperkalemia)

Pharmaceutical

1. Digitalis
2. Beta-adrenergic blockers
3. Quinidine
4. Procainamide
5. Dipyridamole

Pathologic

1. Ischemia

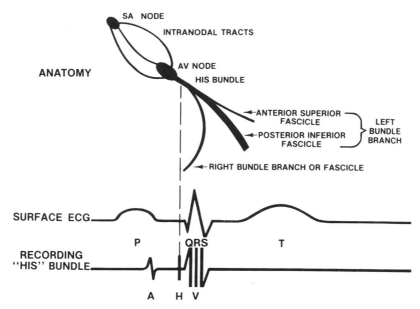

Figure 1. The anatomy of the specialized conducting tissue of the heart and a simultaneous surface and intracardiac electrocardiogram.

2. Infarction
3. Degeneration

SICK SINUS SYNDROME

Patients with conduction delays in and around the sinus and AV nodes manifest a variety of electrocardiographic abnormalities that have been grouped together and referred to as the sick sinus syndrome. The following abnormalities may appear:

Sick sinus
Sluggish sinus node
Lazy sinus node
Sinoatrial syncope
Inadequate sinus mechanism
Bradycardia-tachycardia syndrome

These patients present with a variety of dysrhythmias: (1) persistent, unexplained sinus bradycardia, (2) severe sinus bradycardia associated with hypersensitivity of the carotid sinus, (3) inability of the sinus node to resume firing after cessation of paroxysmal tachycardia or cessation of atrial pacing, or following electrical cardioversion, (4) episodic sinus arrest, and (5) marked sinus bradycardia alternating with tachycardia. The last has been variously referred to as the bradycardia-tachycardia syndrome, tachycardia-bradycardia syndrome, or tachy-brady syndrome. Not infrequently, patients with the tachy-brady syndrome are found to have frequent premature atrial beats, short runs of tachycardia, and periods of apparent SA node arrest (probably SA node exit block), with an inadequate escape mechanism (Fig. 2). Another common sequence in patients with the tachy-brady syndrome is as follows: The patient will enter with a tachycardia, such as atrial fibrillation, with a rapid ventricular response, but severe bradycardia results when therapeutic doses of digitalis are administered in an effort to slow the ventricular response.

The most frequently recognized symptoms of the sick sinus

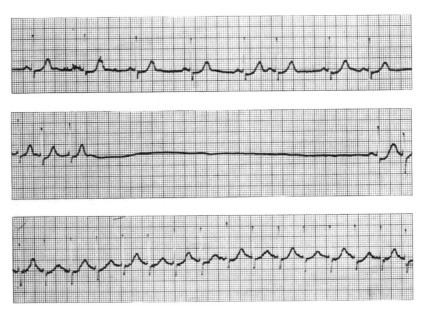

Figure 2. Leads of an electrocardiographic Holter monitor from a patient with a variety of the sick sinus syndrome. The recordings are not continuous. *Top:* Sinus rhythm with premature atrial beats. *Middle:* Sinus rhythm interrupted by a 5.5 second interval of sinus arrest without escape beats. *Bottom:* Supraventricular tachycardia.

syndrome are dizziness, giddiness, and syncope, with or without convulsions. Since the hemodynamic result of the sick sinus syndrome is hypoperfusion of the brain, this syndrome should be suspect in any patient with personality changes, irritability, fleeting memory losses, generalized weakness or fatigue, intermittent slurred speech, or sleeping difficulties. The sick sinus syndrome obviously must be differentiated from transient cerebral ischemic attacks. Hypoperfusion of the heart can exacerbate congestive heart failure and angina pectoris. Palpitation is another symptom that should make one consider the sick sinus syndrome. At first, the association of tachycardia and bradycardia seems a paradox. However, it is now the consensus that paroxysmal atrial tachycardia, atrial flutter, and junctional (nodal) and ventricular tachycardia are all re-entrant arrhythmia and thus require areas of delayed conduction for initiation and maintenance. Therefore, the same abnormality is responsible for both the tachycardia and the bradycardia.

One third of the patients with the sick sinus syndrome have associated conduction defects in the AV node or the trifascicular ventricular conduction system. Figure 3 is the ECG from an

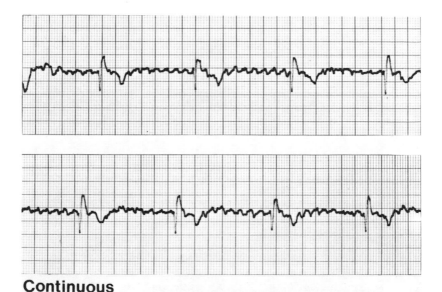

Continuous

Figure 3. A continuous electrocardiogram from a monitor lead. It reveals atrial fibrillation with a regular ventricular response.

ELECTROCARDIOGRAPHIC CONDUCTION DEFECTS 125

elderly man on no medications. The fact that the ventricular response rate is slow and regular in spite of atrial fibrillation suggests complete block at the AV node. This was confirmed by a His's bundle recording (Fig. 4).

The diagnosis of the sick sinus syndrome is made by documenting the electrocardiographic abnormality during symptoms. This usually requires prolonged monitoring. Because of the intermittent nature of the problem, the diagnosis is often difficult, especially in the early stages. Therefore, several provocative tests have been developed, including atropine injection, isoproterenol infusion, and atrial pacing studies. None of these tests are completely satisfactory because of the number of false-positive and negative results, but atropine infusion and atrial pacing have some clinical value.

When 1 to 2 mg atropine is given intravenously to normal in-

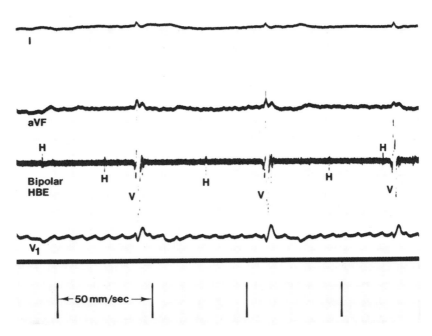

Figure 4. Simultaneous surface and intracardiac electrocardiogram from the same patient whose electrocardiogram was shown in Figure 3. *Top to bottom:* Lead I, lead aVF, bipolar His's bundle electrograph (HBE), and lead V$_1$. The recording speed is 50 mm/sec.

dividuals, the heart rate increases to 100 beats per minute or more. If atropine fails to increase a slow sinus rhythm to 90 beats per minute, the sick sinus syndrome should be suspected.

The recovery time of the sinus nodes is measured following the sudden cessation of rapid atrial pacing. A pacing catheter is used to increase the atrial rate to 120 to 140 beats per minute for 3 to 4 minutes. Atrial pacing is then abruptly terminated. In some patients with the sick sinus syndrome, this results in prolonged and at times symptomatic asystolic intervals before the junctional tissue (around the AV node) resumes discharging, i.e., recovery. If positive, the test is helpful, but lacks sensitivity. Other more sophisticated tests, (e.g., measuring or calculating sinoatrial conduction times by using premature atrial stimulation) also lack sensitivity.

My current recommendation is as follows. In those patients in whom the abnormality is suspected, a detailed review of drug history is made to eliminate possible aggravation of a minor abnormality by drugs, such as beta-adrenergic blockers or excessive amounts of digitalis. Recently it has been shown that the centrally acting antihypertensive medicines, such as alpha-methyldopa, can produce or aggravate the tendency toward the sick sinus syndrome. If the patient is not taking drugs, an atropine challenge should be given (if there is no contraindication). A normal response of the heart rate to atropine should be reassuring to the anesthesiologist. If the response is abnormal, cardiologic consultation should be sought to consider placing a temporary pacemaker for atrial pacing studies and for prophylaxis during surgery.

AV NODAL CONDUCTION DELAYS

Conduction delay in the AV node is manifest by first degree heart block (Fig. 5), i.e., simple prolongation of the PR interval. If one or more impulses from the atrium are completely blocked at the AV node, but some impulses are conducted, second degree heart block is said to be present. Mobitz Type I or Wenckebach phenomenon is manifested by a PR interval that progressively increases until a beat is not conducted. The PR interval of the next conducted beat is shorter than the PR interval of the beat just before the dropped beat. This type of second degree block almost always occurs in the AV node. In Mobitz Type II

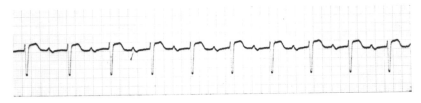

Figure 5. Electrocardiogram showing sinus rhythm and first-degree heart block.

second degree atrioventricular block, the block occurs below the AV node. If none of the atrial impulses result in ventricular activation, then third degree heart block is said to be present. If block occurs only at the AV node and the ventricular conduction system is normal, the QRS configuration is normal.

Block at the AV node may occur because of increased vagal stimulation and decreased sympathetic stimulation (for practical purposes, there is no parasympathetic innervation of the ventricles). Thus, conduction through the AV node is influenced by reflexes as well as by drugs.

Conduction delay or block may also occur because of ischemia of the AV node. Since the major blood supply of the AV node comes from a branch of the right coronary artery in 90 percent of individuals, occlusion of the right coronary artery (usually producing an inferior myocardial infarction) can result in transient heart block.

Fibrosis and degeneration of the AV node tissue are common causes of conduction delay. If the pathology is degeneration or "fibrosis from within," this is referred to as Lenegre's disease. Since the aortic annulus is in close proximity to the conducting system, calcification of the aortic annulus (as may occur in patients with aortic valve disease) may result in encroachment and fibrosis of the conduction system. This "fibrosis from without" is referred to as Lev's disease.

Block at the AV node is not quite as serious as block below the AV node, as the junctional escape rate is faster and the escaping pacemaker more reliable. Many individuals with congenital complete heart block do well for years. Block occurring below the AV node carries a very poor prognosis as the escape rate is slow and undependable.

Patients with second or third degree heart block should have the protection of a transvenous pacemaker during anesthesia.

Patients with first-degree heart block and a normal QRS complex usually do not develop problems. However, the anesthesiologist should rule out digitalis or other drug excess. The response to atropine may be undesirable. Some patients will have first-degree heart block at slow or normal heart rates, but do not conduct every beat with the increased atrial rate secondary to atropine. This occurs in patients with relatively intact SA nodes (and thus the expected increase in sinus rate with atropine) and abnormal AV nodes. Other patients with first-degree heart block secondary to increased vagal effect may normalize conduction with atropine. Patients with significant first-degree heart block who are to receive atropine as a preoperative medication should have this given only with electrocardiographic monitoring.

VENTRICULAR CONDUCTION DEFECTS

The specialized conduction tissue of the ventricles can be functionally and probably anatomically considered to be trifascicular

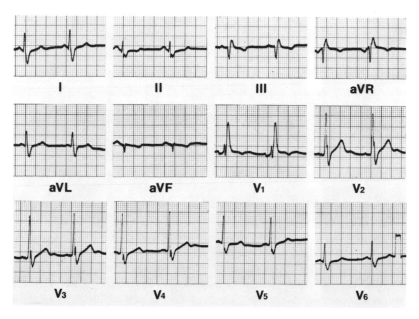

Figure 6. Standard 12-lead electrocardiogram showing a right bundle branch block. Notice the broad S wave in lead I and the R' in lead V₁.

in nature (Fig. 1). The three fascicles are the right bundle branch, the anterior superior division of the left bundle branch, and the posterior inferior division of the left bundle branch.

Complete block of the right bundle branch results in the classic electrocardiographic pattern of right bundle branch block (RBBB) (Fig. 6). Complete block of the left anterior superior division of the left bundle results in left axis deviation (LAD). Complete block of the left posterior inferior division of the left bundle results in right axis deviation (RAD). As illustrated in Figure 7, axis deviation results only from blocks in the fascicles of the left bundle and not from block of the right bundle. The electrocardiographic features of bifascicular block are right bundle branch block with left axis deviation (RBBB and LAD) (Fig. 8), right bundle branch block with right axis deviation (RBBB and RAD) (Fig. 9), and left bundle branch block (LBBB).

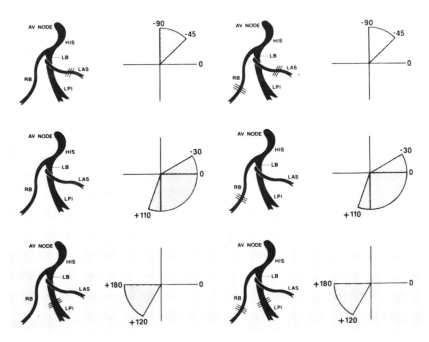

Figure 7. A schematic illustration of the Av node and the specialized conducting system of the ventricles with a schematic illustration of the frontal plane axis. The three hashed lines indicate complete block. The darker areas indicate the resultant axis.

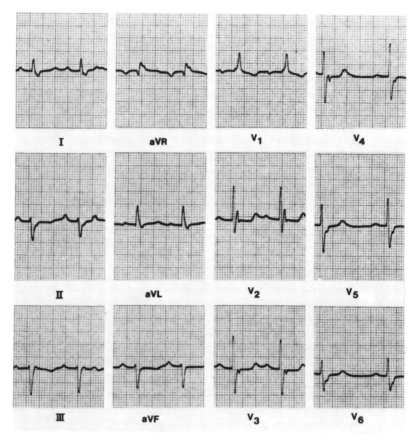

Figure 8. Standard 12-lead electrocardiogram showing right bundle branch block and left axis deviation.

Recognition of bifascicular block is important, since it is a precursor of complete heart block. The relationship between fascicular block, bundle branch block, and complete heart block is illustrated in Figure 10. However, the time interval between bifascicular block and complete heart block varies from minutes to decades, and the object of the preoperative evaluation is to determine whether the progression is likely to occur with the stress of anesthesia and surgery. To make this decision, one has to determine the status of the third fascicle. Recall that conduction abnormalities may result in slight, moderate, or severe conduction delays or complete block. If there is complete block of

ELECTROCARDIOGRAPHIC CONDUCTION DEFECTS   131

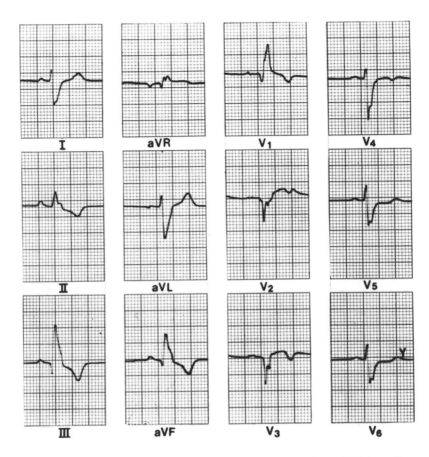

Figure 9. Standard 12-lead electrocardiogram revealing right bundle branch block and right axis deviation.

the right bundle branch and left anterior superior fascicle, and a delay in conduction via the posterior inferior fascicle, the ECG will show a RBBB, LAD, and first-degree heart block, i.e., a prolonged PR interval (Fig. 8). However, this PR prolongation may result if the delay is either in the AV node or in the third fascicle. The only way to determine this is to do His's bundle recordings. Referring back to Figure 1, if the delay is in the AV node, the AH interval will be prolonged, and if the delay is in the fascicular conduction system, the HV interval will be prolonged. All old ECGs of the patient should be reviewed, as previous conduction

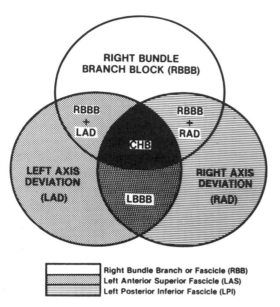

Figure 10. Relation of conduction defects to bifascicular and complete heart block.

delays in the third fascicle may have been present on an old ECG, which would indicate a diagnosis of trifascicular block. For example, a patient with a previous right bundle branch block who now has left bundle branch block surely has trifascicular disease.

A patient with left bundle branch block and first-degree heart block (prolonged PR) has block of the left bundle (or its two fascicles), but again, the prolonged PR interval may be from delay either through the AV node or the right bundle. A His's bundle recording revealing a prolonged HV interval would indicate concomitant involvement of the third fascicles. Figure 11 is a His's bundle recording from a patient with LBBB. The electrocardiographic manifestations of problems of fascicular conduction are outlined in Table 1.

This brings us to the important questions. Should all patients with potential trifascicular block (RBBB, LAD, and first-degree heart block; RBBB, RAD, and first-degree heart block; or LBB and first-degree heart block) receive prophylactic pacemakers prior to surgery and should they have His's bundle recording to

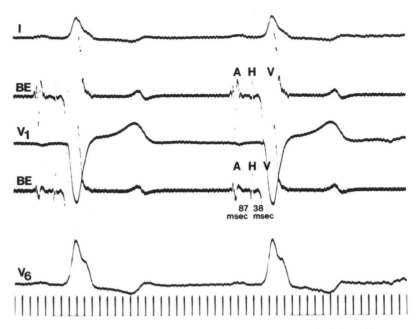

Figure 11. His's bundle recording from a patient with left bundle branch block. *Top to bottom:* Lead I, bipolar intracardiac electrode, lead V_1, bipolar intracardiac electrode, and lead V_6. The AH and the HV intervals are normal.

determine whether a prolonged HV interval is present? There is very little objective information on these questions. Two retrospective reports on small groups of patients with bifascicular block, who underwent surgery, suggest that the chance of developing complete heart block is small. Their recommendations

Table 1. Electrocardiographic Manifestations of Conduction Delays or Blocks

Fascicular	Bifascicular	Incomplete Trifascicular	Complete Trifascicular
RBBB	RBBB + LAD	RBBB + LAD + 1° HB	CHB
RAD	RBBB + RAD	RBBB + RAD + 1° HB	
LAD	LBBB	LBBB + 1° HB	
		Masquerading BBB	
		Alternating BBB	

are that those patients be closely monitored during and after surgery, but that prophylactic pacemakers are not indicated.

There are three large studies addressing the question of whether a permanent pacemaker should be placed in individuals with RBBB, LAD, and prolonged HV intervals as determined by His's bundle recording. The authors of these studies conclude that if such patients are not symptomatic, prophylactic pacemakers are not indicated. However, if symptoms are present that are not caused by other disease processes (such as ventricular arrhythmias or postural hypotension), permanent pacemakers are indicated.

Patients with masquerading bundle branch block, i.e., left bundle branch pattern in lead I and right bundle branch block pattern in lead V_1, or vice versa, should have a pacemaker. Likewise, patients with alternating bundle branch block, i.e., some beats conducted with right bundle branch pattern and some with left bundle branch pattern, should have a pacemaker.

SUMMARY

Prophylactic pacemakers should be recommended for all preoperative patients with second- and third-degree heart block, regardless of whether the block is in the AV node or the trifascicular conduction system. Symptomatic patients with potential for trifascicular block should also have a transvenous pacemaker. Those without symptoms should be monitored during anesthesia and the postoperative recovery period.

ACKNOWLEDGEMENTS

The author greatly appreciates the secretarial assistance of Miss Ann C. Vallefuoco and the services of Biomedical Communications of the Arizona Health Sciences Center.

BIBLIOGRAPHY

1. Berg, G. R., and Kotler, M. N.: *The significance of bilateral bundle branch block in the preoperative patient.* Chest 59:62, 1971.
2. Dhingra, R. C., Bauernfeind, R., Swiryn, S., et al.: *Evaluation and management of conduction disease.* Cardiovasc. Med. May:493, 1978.

3. Rios, J. C., Fletcher, R. M., Ewy, G. A., et al.: *Electrocardiographic precursors of complete heart block.* Ariz. Med. 30:164, 1973.
4. Kulbertus, H. E.: *The magnitude of risk of developing complete heart block in patients with LAD-RBBB.* Am. Heart J. 86:278, 1973.
5. McAnulty, J. H., and Rahimtoola, S. H.: *Sudden death and high risk bundle branch block.* Cardiovasc. Med. July:711, 1978.
6. McAnulty, J. H., Rahimtoola, S. H., Murphy, E. S., et al.: *A prospective study of sudden death in "high-risk" bundle branch block.* N. Engl. J. Med. 299:209, 1978.
7. Scheinman, M. M., Peters, R. W., Modin, G., et al: *Prognostic value of infranodal conduction time in patients with chronic bundle branch block.* Circulation 56:240, 1977.
8. Venkataraman, K., Madias, J. E., and Hood, W. B., Jr.: *Indications for prophylactic preoperative insertion of pacemakers in patients with right bundle branch block and left anterior hemiblock.* Chest 68:501, 1975.

DIAGNOSIS AND THERAPY OF PERIOPERATIVE ARRHYTHMIAS*

John L. Atlee, III, M.D.

Dr. Atlee brings to light the common arrhythmias associated with general anesthesia. Probable mechanisms, pathophysiology, and therapy are discussed. Tables summarizing various arrhythmias and treatment have been added for clarity for the practitioner. Drug interactions as causes of these events are discussed. It is of historical note that the first defined drug interaction, that of epinephrine and hydrocarbon anesthetics, which produces ventricular arrhythmias, occurs in an anesthetic setting.

Burnell R. Brown, Jr.

*Supported by NIH Grant 1 R23 GM25064–01.

The treatment of cardiac arrhythmias can no longer be based on clinical empiricism. Physiologists have introduced microelectrode and voltage clamping techniques, the use of which has led to a more complete understanding of the cellular and subcellular mechanisms responsible for arrhythmias and antiarrhythmic drug action.[1-4] The application of cardiac electrophysiologic techniques, including His's bundle electrocardiography and atrial or ventricular extrastimulation, has provided clinical verification of postulated arrhythmic mechanisms and improved the efficacy of arrhythmic management.[5-8]

Cardiac arrhythmias are considered disorders of automaticity, conduction, or both.[9] Two forms of automaticity may be involved in production of arrhythmia: (1) abnormalities in diastolic (phase 4) depolarization, associated with sinus node and subsidiary or latent pacemaker foci; and (2) the recently described mechanism of oscillatory afterpotentials, or as it is also referred to, triggered automaticity.[10, 11] The latter is currently regarded as the mechanism for many arrhythmias caused by digitalis excess, rather than enhanced phase 4 automaticity, as was formerly postulated.[10, 11] Since different ionic events are responsible for the two forms of automaticity,[3, 12] they may respond differently to drugs or other interventions used to treat arrhythmias. At the present time, it is not known how anesthetics affect the second of the two mechanisms of automaticity.

Conduction disorders can also be a cause of arrhythmias. Impaired conduction may be responsible for first-, second- or third-degree AV block. Impaired conduction is also necessary for arrhythmias caused by re-entry of excitation.[13]

The decision to treat an arrhythmia is based on proper recognition and observation of hemodynamic consequences. An understanding of mechanisms is required if appropriate antiarrhythmic drug or electrical therapy is going to be used. Arrhythmias warrant treatment in the clinical setting when they: (1) interfere adversely with hemodynamics; (2) upset a favorable balance between myocardial oxygen supply and demand; or (3) predispose the patient to life-threatening arrhythmias, such as ventricular tachycardia or fibrillation. The first consideration in the treatment of arrhythmias, especially in the perioperative setting, is to remove the precipitating cause or causes.

CAUSES OF ARRHYTHMIA DURING ANESTHESIA

It is probable that many of the cardiac arrhythmias seen by anesthetists are related to agents or techniques being used. Chief among the causes during anesthesia (and postanesthetic recovery) are *hypoxia, hypercapnia,* and *hypocapnia.* In most instances, correcting the inappropriate ventilatory pattern and selecting the proper inspired oxygen tension will bring the blood gases into a more normal range, thereby restoring normal cardiac rhythm. Attempts should always be made to improve oxygenation and ventilation before considering other types of treatment. Hypoxia is too well known as a cause of arrhythmias to deserve additional comment. Hypercapnia causes acidosis, provokes the release of endogenous catecholamines, and may trigger ventricular arrhythmias, especially in the presence of hydrocarbon inhalation agents.[14-17] Hypocapnia causes alkalosis and compensatory serum electrolytic shifts, which may predispose the patient to arrhythmias. There can be a decrease in the serum potassium level of as much as 0.5 mEq per liter for every 10-torr fall in arterial pCO_2.[18] Hypocapnic hypokalemia could be particularly dangerous in patients receiving digitalis or potassium-wasting diuretics.

Anesthetic agents themselves can cause arrhythmias. Halothane, methoxyflurane, and probably enflurane cause a dose-related depression of sinus node automaticity.[19] Suppression of the dominant (sinus) pacemaker is accompanied by the emergence of subsidiary pacemakers found in the AV junctional tissues. Smith and coworkers have demonstrated in healthy, human volunteers anesthetized with enflurane an approximate 50 percent incidence of AV junctional arrhythmias.[20] The loss of atrial function accompanying these arrhythmias resulted in hemodynamically significant reductions in cardiac output, stroke volume, and mean arterial pressure.[20] Recently, these same observations have been extended to halothane.[21] Thus, junctional arrhythmias, which most anesthesiologists consider benign relative to rhythm disturbances such as supraventricular tachycardia or ventricular arrhythmias, have the potential for adversely affecting hemodynamics and are of special concern in patients with compromised cardiovascular function. A sudden fall in blood pressure in the absence of obvious causes, such as major blood loss, should alert the anesthetist to the possibility of an AV junctional arrhythmia.

It is well known that hydrocarbon anesthetics may *sensitize the myocardium* to the arrhythmogenic effects of endogenous or exogenous cathecholamines.[22] Although enflurane appears to be less sensitizing than halothane,[23] it is recommended that no more than 10 ml of a 1:100,000 solution of epinephrine be injected over a 10-minute period, or a total of 30 ml in 1 hour during anesthesia with any hydrocarbon anesthetic agent.[22] Although limits for the safe administration of epinephrine during anesthesia with nitrous oxide and narcotics have not been established, I have not observed ventricular arrhythmias when the preceding recommended limits of dosage for epinephrine were adhered to.

Arrhythmias are often associated with *tracheal intubation.* The cause for these arrhythmias is widely debated.[24] In most patients the arrhythmias are relatively benign, since they do not seriously alter hemodynamic function, and can usually be terminated by adequate ventilation of the patient or by deepening the level of anesthesia. In patients with severely compromised cardiac function, coronary artery disease, hypertension, or hyperthyroidism, arrhythmias related to tracheal intubation may not be so innocuous. For such patients at risk, I recommend establishing an adequate level of anesthesia before endotracheal intubation, rather than the customary "sleep dose" of thiopental. The level of anesthesia should be compatible with maintenance of adequate cardiac output. In some borderline or overtly hypertensive patients, I have used small doses of propranolol (1.0 to 2.0 mg I.V., 10 to 15 minutes prior to the induction of anesthesia) as a prophylactic measure against arrhythmias and untoward hypertensive sequelae that are related to endotracheal intubation. This practice is based on the findings of Prys-Roberts and coworkers, who have observed the effectiveness of specific beta-receptor blockade in attenuating the hypertensive cardiovascular responses and arrhythmias attendant to intubation.[25]

Administration of *succinylcholine* may be associated with arrhythmias. This is particularly likely following repeated doses[24] and probably occurs because choline produced from the hydrolysis of succinylcholine by pseudocholinesterase sensitizes the heart to subsequent doses of succinylcholine.[26] Arrhythmias are seen more often in children than adults[24]; this may relate to the common practice of using thiopental, which prevents succinylcholine-related arrhythmias,[26] for the induction of anesthesia in adults but not in children.[24] It is well recognized that life-threatening ventricular arrhythmias are associated with the use of succinylcholine in patients with severe burns,[27-29] extensive muscular damage,[30-32] extensive denervation of skeletal muscle,[33-38] and in patients with peritonitis.[39] The mechanism responsible for these arrhythmias involves the sudden release of large amounts of potassium into the circulation from damaged tissues or denervated muscle. While in theory the prior administration of a nondepolarizing muscle relaxant (*d*-tubocurarine) might be protective against arrhythmias, in practice the protection afforded is not always reliable[33] and therefore cannot be recommended. Finally, the administration of succinylcholine to fully digitalized patients may be followed by ventricular arrhythmias.[40] It appears that the prior administration of *d*-tubocurarine will prevent this response.[40, 41]

There are many specific autonomic causes of arrhythmias during anesthesia and surgery.[24] *Traction reflexes,* such as those involving hollow viscera or extrinsic ocular muscles, and *stimulation of the central nervous system* should be recognized as potential causes of arrhythmias that can be avoided or minimized by cooperative surgical and anesthetic management. For example, Schwartz has found that the incidence of the oculocardiac reflex, which results from pressure on the eyeball or traction on the extraocular muscles, can be significantly reduced by retrobulbar block or by the parenteral administration of atropine.[42] However, I have found that arrhythmias or bradycardia resulting from this reflex are easily abolished by temporarily stopping the surgical manipulation. Subsequent stimulation is usually not accompanied by arrhythmias or as marked a bradycardia.

Other causes of arrhythmias during anesthesia and surgery, including *electrolyte* and *acid-base disturbances,* or *digitalis intoxication,* are largely avoidable in properly prepared patients. Prime offenders in these categories are hypokalemia, seen in many patients on chronic diuretic therapy, and hyperkalemia, associated with renal failure. Hypokalemia, hypomagnesemia, or hypercalcemia may precipitate digitalis toxicity and arrhythmias in a patient who was not overtly toxic beforehand. I prefer not to anesthetize patients with renal failure who have serum potassium levels greater than 5.5 mEq/liter. In emergencies, when the potassium level cannot be lowered by such conventional forms of treatment as potassium-exchange resins or dialysis, I administer calcium chloride, sodium bicarbonate, glucose, and insulin to acutely lower the serum potassium to more acceptable levels.

Clearly there are many potential causes of arrhythmias in the perioperative setting. Most of these can be avoided by adequate preoperative assessment and skillful intraoperative management of anesthetized patients. Some causes of arrhythmias may be related to the surgical procedure. Recognition of these by both the anesthetist and surgeon will often reduce the incidence or severity of the potential rhythm disturbances. Regardless of how well an anesthetic is conducted, some arrhythmias will occur that require treatment, or, following preoperative assessment, may modify the contemplated plan of anesthetic management. The following sections consider the most common clinically encountered arrhythmias and their management and summarize the actions, indications, dosage, and major side effects of drugs used to treat arrhythmias.

CLASSIFICATION AND MANAGEMENT OF ARRHYTHMIAS

Cardiac rhythm disturbance will be considered in four principal categories: isolated premature beats, bradyarrhythmias, tachyarrhythmias, and AV conduction block. While this is a simpler classification of arrhythmias than that likely to be used by a specialist in electrocardiography, it is well suited to the needs of the anesthetist, who frequently may have neither the means nor the time to distinguish between complex rhythm disturbances. Some of the more common arrhythmias found within each category are listed in Table 1. I have summarized in Table 2 the principal modalities of treatment for each type of rhythm disturbance. Table 3 lists the actions, indications, dosages, and major side effects of the drugs commonly used in the perioperative setting.

A more detailed discussion of the recognition and management of arrhythmias within each category follows.

Table 1. Classification of Cardiac Arrhythmias.

Premature Beats	Bradyarrhythmias	Tachyarrhythmias	AV Block
Atrial	Sinus bradycardia	Sinus tachycardia	First-degree
AV junctional	Sinoatrial block	Paroxysmal atrial tachycardia	Second-degree
Ventricular	Sinus arrhythmia	Atrial tachycardia with block	Mobitz I
	Junctional bradycardia	Multifocal atrial tachycardia	Mobitz II
	Indioventricular bradycardia	Atrial flutter	Advanced
	Wandering atrial pacemaker	Atrial fibrillation	Third-degree
	Isorhythmic dissociation	Ventricular tachycardia	Bundle branch
		Ventricular fibrillation	Hemiblock
			Anterior
			Posterior

Table 2. Summary of Principal Treatment Modalities for Perioperative Arrhythmias.

Category	Type	Treatment
Premature beats	Atrial	None usually; treat cause.
Premature beats	AV junctional	None usually; treat cause.
Premature beats	Ventricular	Treat cause; lidocaine, phenytoin.
Bradyarrhythmias	Sinus bradycardia	Treat cause; atropine; ephedrine or mephentermine (high spinal block); isoproterenol (if due to propranolol).
Bradyarrhythmias	Sinoatrial block	Treat cause (e.g., digitalis toxicity); atropine; electronic pacemaker.
Bradyarrhythmias	Sinus arrest	Same as for sinoatrial block.
Bradyarrhythmias	Sinus arrhythmia	None usually; symptomatic sick sinus syndrome; atropine.
Bradyarrhythmias	Junctional bradycardia	Treat cause (e.g., anesthetic-related, digitalis toxicity); electronic pacemaker.
Bradyarrhythmias	Idioventricular bradycardia	Treat cause (e.g., digitalis toxicity); electronic pacemaker.
Bradyarrhythmias	Wandering atrial pacemaker	Treat cause (e.g., anesthetic-related); ephedrine; mephentermine if circulation compromised.
Bradyarrhythmias	Isorhythmic dissociation	Same as for wandering atrial pacemaker.
Tachyarrhythmias	Sinus tachycardia	Treat cause (e.g., light anesthesia, blood loss); propranolol for patient with signs of myocardial ischemia.
Tachyarrhythmias	Paroxysmal S-V tachycardia	Carotid sinus massage; Valsalva maneuver; edrophonium; neostigmine; methoxamine; phenylephrine; digitalis; propranolol; DC cardioversion; electronic pacing (overdrive suppression).

Tachyarrhythmias	Atrial tachycardia with block	Frequent sign of digitalis toxicity, treat if cause (phenytoin; occasionally lidocaine is effective); cardioversion (if not due to digitalis), but disturbance usually recurs.
Tachyarrhythmias	Multifocal atrial tachycardia	Same as for atrial tachycardia with block.
Tachyarrhythmias	Atrial flutter	Digitalis; cardioversion; quinidine; procainamide.
Tachyarrhythmias	Atrial fibrillation	Same as atrial flutter.
Tachyarrhythmias	Ventricular tachycardia	Treat cause (e.g., digitalis toxicity); lidocaine, phenytoin; cardioversion.
Tachyarrhythmias	Ventricular fibrillation	Cardioversion (epinephrine to facilitate); lidocaine, phenytoin to prevent recurrences.
AV block	First-degree	No specific treatment usually; atropine.
AV block	Second-degree, Mobitz I	None usually; treat cause (e.g., digitalis toxicity); isoproterenol; atropine; rarely, electronic pacemaker.
AV block	Second-degree, Mobitz II or advanced	Permanent electronic pacemaker (drugs usually ineffective).
AV block	Third-degree, complete	Permanent electronic pacemaker (except in some cases of congenital complete AV block).
AV block	Bundle branch	None for isolated right bundle branch block; electronic pacing for symptomatic left bundle branch block or left bundle branch block associated with second degree AV block.
AV block	Hemiblock, anterior or posterior	None for monofascicular block or asymptomatic bifascicular block; electronic pacemaker for symptomatic bifascicular block or bifascicular block with second-degree AV block.

Table 3. Summary of Indications, Actions, Dosages, and Major Side Effects of Drugs Used in the Treatment of Cardiac Arrhythmias in the Perioperative Setting.

Drug	Action	Indications	Dosage	Side Effects
Atropine	Anticholinergic (muscarinic)	1. Sinus bradycardia 2. Sinoatrial block 3. Bradyarrhythmias, AV block 2° reflex increase vagal tone	1. Adults: 0.4–0.6 mg I.V. (vagal blocking dose 1.0–3.0 mg I.V.) 2. Children: 0.10 mg/10 kg body wt. I.V.	1. CNS stimulation (excitement delirium) 2. Initial cardiac slowing 3. Tachycardia 4. Increased myocardial oxygen consumption 5. Arrhythmias when used during anesthesia
Digoxin	Slow AV conduction	Slow ventricular rate: 1. Atrial flutter/ fibrillation 2. Atrial tachy-arrhythmias not responsive to carotid sinus massage	1. Adults: 0.75–1.5 mg I.V. for full digitalization (loading dose ½ digitalizing dose) 2. Children: 30–50 mcg/kg I.V. for full digitalization (loading dose ½ digitalizing dose)	1. Ventricular arrhythmias 2. AV block
Edrophonium	Anticholinesterase	Paroxysmal atrial tachycardia	10 mg I.V.	1. Bradycardia 2. AV block 3. Increased pharyngeal secretions

Drug	Classification	Indication	Dose	Complications
Ephedrine	Vasopressor (mixed alpha- and beta-adrenergic agonist; indirect and direct actions)	Bradycardia and hypotension related to: 1. High spinal block 2. Deep level of anesthesia	5–10 mg I.V.	1. Tachycardia 2. Hypertension
Epinephrine	Vasopressor (mixed alpha- and beta-adrenergic agonist; direct action)	To facilitate electrical conversion of heart following cardiac arrest	0.1–1.0 mg I.V. (central line) or intracardiac	1. Tachycardia 2. Hypertension 3. Ventricular arrhythmias
Isoproterenol	Vasopressor (beta-adrenergic agonist; direct action)	Bradycardia AV block	1. 0.1 mg I.V. 2. Continuous infusion (1.0 mg in 250 ml NSS)	1. Tachycardia 2. Ventricular arrhythmias
Lidocaine	Antiarrhythmic	Ventricular arrhythmias	1. Loading: 100–200 mg I.V. 2. Infusion: 1.0 g in 250 ml NSS (20–30 mcg/kg/min)	1. Seizures 2. Ventricular acceleration in atrial flutter/fibrillation
Mephentermine	Vasopressor (mixed alpha- and beta-adrenergic agonist; indirect and direct actions)	Bradycardia and hypotension related to: 1. High spinal block 2. Deep levels of anesthesia	5–10 mg I.V.	1. Tachycardia 2. Hypertension
Methoxamine	Vasopressor (alpha-adrenergic agonist)	Paroxysmal atrial tachycardia	5–10 mg I.V.	1. Hypertension 2. AV block (reflex) 3. Bradycardia (reflex)
Neostigmine	Anticholinesterase	Paroxysmal atrial tachycardia	1.0 mg I.V.	1. Bradycardia 2. AV block 3. Increased pharyngeal secretions

Table 3. Continued.

Drug	Action	Indications	Dosage	Side Effects
Neosynephrine	Vasopressor (alpha-adrenergic agonist)	Paroxysmal atrial tachycardia	0.1–1.0 mg I.V.	1. Hypertension 2. AV block (reflex) 3. Bradycardia (reflex)
Phenytoin (diphenyl-hydantoin)	Antiarrhythmic	1. Digitalis induced ventricular arrhythmias; may be effective in some supraventricular arrhythmias due to digitalis 2. Given prior to electrical conversion for patients with atrial flutter/fibrillation on digitalis	50–100 mg I.V. repeated every 10–15 minutes until clinical therapeutic effect observed, or maximum dose of 10–15 mg/kg administered	1. Respiratory arrest 2. SA nodal arrest 3. AV block
Propranolol	Antiarrhythmic (beta-adrenergic blocker)	1. To slow ventricular response in supraventricular arrhythmias 2. In control of ventricular arrhythmias, when electrical conversion contraindicated because of digitalis toxicity	0.25–3.0 mg I.V. (divided doses)	1. Myocardial depression: hypotension 2. AV block 3. Bradycardia 4. Bronchospasm

Isolated Premature Beats

After sinus tachycardia, premature beats of supraventricular or ventricular origin are the most common disturbances of normal cardiac rhythm seen in the perioperative setting. Isolated premature beats may arise from any portion of the atria, AV junctional tissues (including the AV node), or ventricles. Examples of such beats are shown in Figures 1 and 2. While their isolated

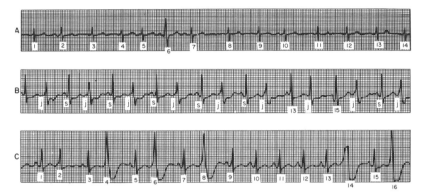

Figure 1. Premature beats of atrial, AV junctional, and ventricular origin. *A*, Surface electrocardiographic lead II from a 62-year-old male undergoing aortocoronary bypass surgery. Beats 1, 3, 4, 8, 9, and 11–14 are of probable sinus origin. Beats 2, 5–7, and 10 are premature atrial beats. Beat 6 is associated with aberrant (ventricular) conduction. *B*, Surface electrocardiographic lead II from 38-year-old female undergoing laparoscopy for tubal banding. Junctional premature beats (j) are coupled (bigeminy) with each sinus beat (s), although the P waves associated with the thirteenth and fifteenth QRS complexes may not be of sinus origin but rather have been caused by a wandering atrial pacemaker. Junctional premature beats are associated with aberrant conduction. This arrhythmia was recorded during tracheal intubation. *C*, Surface electrocardiographic lead II from a 67-year-old male undergoing exploratory laparotomy. Arrhythmias were recorded during laryngoscopy prior to intubation of trachea. Beats 1, 3, 5, 7, 9–13, and 15 are of sinus origin. The second beat appears to be a junctional premature beat. Beats 4, 6, 8, 14, and 16 are probably ventricular premature beats, although in the absence of compensatory pauses, they could be supraventricular premature beats with a marked degree of aberrant conduction.

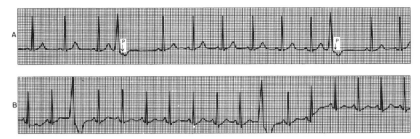

Figure 2. Premature ventricular beats recorded (electrocardiographic lead II) during laryngoscopy and tracheal intubation in a 20-year-old female juvenile diabetic undergoing elective sterilization. *A*, Ventricular premature beats followed by a compensatory pause. Note the P wave inscribed within the ST segment of the premature beats. *B*, Ventricular premature beats not followed by a compensatory pause. The timing of the premature beats coincides with that of the sinus beat. The basic mechanism is sinus tachycardia (100 beats per minute).

occurrence is not necessarily an indication of underlying disease or patient mismanagement, they may frequently be a warning that some physiologic or pharmacologic trespass has occurred. Therefore, the cardinal rule regarding treatment must be to seek and identify the cause. Premature beats do not require specific treatment, except when they are of multifocal origin or occur frequently. The reason for treating frequent, R on T, bigeminal, or multifocal ventricular premature beats is not because of impaired hemodynamics, but because they may be the forerunners of more serious rhythm disturbances, including tachycardia and fibrillation. Frequent or multifocal atrial premature beats may also be the forerunners of tachyarrhythmias (of atrial origin). They are usually not treated, however.

In the operating room it may be difficult to distinguish premature supraventricular beats associated with aberrant ventricular conduction from ventricular ectopic beats. Not only are the usual criteria for determining the origin of premature beats occasionally misleading (Table 4), but also the monitoring leads commonly employed in the perioperative setting may be unreliable for purposes of differentiation. An example is the compensatory pause (the interval between P waves of the beats immediately preceding and following the premature beats is twice the normal PP interval) of ventricular as opposed to supraventricu-

Table 4. Criteria for Determining the Origin of Premature Beats.

Ventricular	Supraventricular
Not preceded by P wave	Preceded by P wave
Compensatory pause	No compensatory pause
Widened QRS complexes with bizarre appearance	If associated with ventricular aberration, less widened QRS complexes that are less bizarre in appearance
T wave in opposite direction of normal T wave	T wave in same direction as normal T wave

lar ectopy (Fig. 2A). Supraventricular beats that are sufficiently premature to be conducted aberrantly may be followed by a compensatory pause if the timing of the normal sinus beat coincides with the QRS complex of the premature beat. In this case, the sinus mechanism is not interfered with, and the next normal beat would appear compensated. Supraventricular premature beats may be associated with some delay in conduction of the next normal beat.[43] Thus the RR interval between the premature and next normal beat is longer than the normal RR interval, but not fully compensated.

An important rule when attempting to determine the origin of premature beats is to look for a P wave preceding the premature beat. It is not present with ventricular ectopy, and not apparent in the case of low junctional premature beats. Low junctional premature beats associated with aberrant ventricular conduction may be next to impossible to differentiate from ventricular premature beats, especially when the junctional beats are followed by a compensatory pause. These beats may require intracardiac conduction studies to determine their origin. Finally, a P wave arising from a nonsinal atrial focus that is responsible for a premature beat may be isoelectric in the monitoring lead selected. This is usually surface lead II. For this reason, the electrocardiographic monitor should give the anesthetist flexibility in the selection of leads. These should include, as a minimum, surface leads I, II, and III; and, preferably, also aVR, aVL, aVF, and V leads. The V lead is used for the detection of myocardial ischemia in tachyarrhythmias. With properly grounded electrocardiographic monitoring equipment, it is possible to substitute an intra-atrial or esophageal lead for the V lead. This will give the clinician the ability to accurately time atrial and ventricular events in arrhythmias that are difficult to interpret. An example of the difficulty that can sometimes be encountered in distinguishing supraventricular from ventricular ectopy is given in Figure 3.

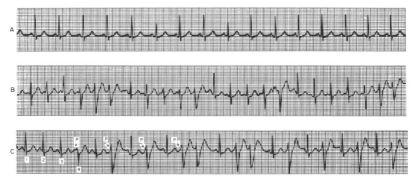

Figure 3. Arrhythmias seen following the injection of epinephrine (6.0 ml 1:200,000 epinephrine in 0.5 percent lidocaine) for surgical hemostasis. Cartilage strut (rib) rhinoplasty performed in a 16-year-old female under enflurane-oxygen anesthesia. A, Sinus rhythm (88 beats per minute) prior to injection of epinephrine (lead II). B, Multifocal atrial tachycardia (heart rate varies between 100 and 150 beats per minute) seen approximately 1 minute following epinephrine. Most beats are associated with varying degrees of aberrant ventricular conduction, and some QRS complexes are sufficiently deformed and bizarre in appearance to be easily mistaken for ventricular premature beats. Note that there are no compensatory pauses, and the T waves remain upright with all beats. C, One minute later, underlying sinus tachycardia (beats 1, 2, and 3) with a rate of approximately 120 beats per minute is seen. Beat 4 is probably of high junctional origin and associated with aberrant ventricular conduction. The remaining nonsinus beats are probably also of junctional origin (note the P wave that deforms each R wave) and associated with more marked aberrant conduction. The rather bizarre QRS complexes and large (upright) T waves could easily be mistaken for ventricular bigeminy or trigeminy. These arrhythmias (B and C) were not associated with increases in the patient's blood pressure (it remained at 140/70). They were not treated and spontaneously subsided within 5 minutes after they first appeared. Arterial blood gas values immediately following the arrhythmias were normal.

ANESTHESIA AND THE PATIENT WITH HEART DISEASE

Premature supraventricular beats, even though they can predispose the patient to supraventricular tachyarrhythmias, are usually not treated. This is because their hemodynamic impact is, in most cases, inconsequential. Should a tachyarrhythmia ensue, the treatment becomes that of the resulting arrhythmia (discussed later). While in theory drugs such as quinidine or procainamide would be effective in the treatment of supraventricular premature beats, their toxicity makes them less than ideal for parenteral use in anesthetized patients. Since both drugs are direct myocardial depressants and vasodilators,[44] their effects may be additive to those of anesthetic agents.

Ventricular premature beats may be normal, but frequently they are iatrogenically imposed by anesthetic misadventure. This implies that the treatment is simple enough: remove the precipitating cause or causes. Occasionally, however, as in surgery for pheochromocytoma or following the excessive use of epinephrine for surgical hemostasis, ventricular premature beats may be persistent or serious enough to warrant treatment. Such is the case if the premature beats are closely coupled to the preceding normal beats (bigeminy or trigeminy); occur in runs of three to five or more (ventricular tachycardia); or are multifocal in origin; or if the R wave of the premature beat falls on the T wave of the preceding normal beat. Lidocaine is the preferred drug for treating premature ventricular beats. Initial therapy consists of an intravenous bolus of 1.0 to 2.0 mg/kg body weight. If arrhythmias recur following initial treatment, a continuous intravenous infusion of lidocaine is indicated. Lidocaine (1000 mg) mixed in 250 ml of normal saline is infused at a rate of 20 to 30 mcg/kg body weight per minute.

Ventricular ectopy resulting from imbalances of serum electrolytes, but requiring immediate therapy, may be temporarily treated with lidocaine while the imbalance is corrected. Ventricular ectopy caused by digitalis excess, or digitalis toxicity provoked by hypokalemia, hypomagnesemia, or hypercalcemia, may not respond to lidocaine. Intravenous phenytoin (diphenylhydantoin) administered intravenously is the drug of choice when the arrhythmia fails to respond to lidocaine. The administration of potassium (or magnesium) to the patient with digitalis toxicity may be therapeutic.

Therapeutic serum concentrations of phenytoin (8 to 16 mcg/ml) can be attained by the slow administration of doses of 50 to 100 mg every 10 to 15 minutes until a therapeutic response is observed, or a maximum dose of 10 to 15 mg/kg body weight has been given.[45, 46] Caution, however, should be used in the intravenous administration of phenytoin, since there is the danger of producing asystole, AV conduction block, or respiratory arrest.[44] Phenytoin should only be used for ventricular arrhythmias related to digitalis excess after lidocaine has proved ineffective. Lidocaine has potentially less harmful effects on cardiac conduction and function of sinus nodes. It is the preferred immediate drug treatment for most ventricular arrhythmias.

Bradyarrhythmias

Bradyarrhythmias include those disturbances of normal heart rhythm, excluding AV conduction block, in which the ventricular response is less than 60 beats per minute in adults; less than 80 beats per minute in children; and less than 100 beats per minute in infants.[43] Sinus bradycardia is the most common of the bradyarrhythmias, but is not in itself an indication of organic or drug-related heart dysfunction. Sinoatrial block occurs when sinus impulses fail to penetrate into and capture the atria. This is another cause of slow heart rates and usually indicates the presence of disordered sinus function or conduction block at the sinoatrial junction. Slow heart rates may also result from such nonsinus mechanisms as AV junctional rhythm or idioventricular rhythm. These two arrhythmias occur when the sinus node is depressed or there is complete AV block. Finally, wandering atrial pacemaker and isorhythmic AV dissociation, which are quite common arrhythmias during anesthesia, may be associated with slow heart rates.

Sinus bradycardia does not require treatment unless it is symptomatic in the awake patient or causes a clinically significant drop in cardiac output and blood pressure in the anesthetized patient. It is frequently related to deep levels of anesthesia. Sinus bradycardia may occur following spinal or epidural anesthesia if the segmental level of block affects the cardiac accelerator nerves (T_1–T_4). Sinus bradycardia caused by deep levels of anesthesia or high sympathetic block can lead to significant hypotension. This is especially true in patients with large deficits in intravascular volume. While other deficits are being corrected, it may be desirable to increase the sinus rate by administering atropine (0.4 to 0.6 mg I.V. for adults; 0.1 mg/10 kg body

weight for children). Ephedrine (5 to 10 mg I.V.) or mephentermine (5 to 10 mg I.V.) may also be used to increase heart rate
and blood pressure. Following these relatively small doses of
atropine, however, there may be an initial reduction in heart rate
caused by central stimulation of vagal centers, peripheral stimulation of parasympathetic receptors, inhibition of acetylcholin-
esterase, effects on the sympathetic nervous system, or by direct
effects on the cardiac pacemaker cells.[47] This parasympathomi-
metic action of atropine is probably responsible for the arrhythmias seen when it is administered to anesthetized patients.[48]
Doses of atropine greater than 0.6 mg I.V. do not cause a significant slowing of the heart rate in most patients.[47, 48] Doses of 1.0
to 3.0 mg I.V. may be required to completely block the cardiac
effects of the vagus.[49] Finally, large doses of atropine should be
used with caution in patients with coronary artery disease, since
they can lead to ischemia or actual infarction.

Periods of *sinus arrest, sinoatrial block,* and *sinus arrhythmia*
may all be responsible for slow heart rates. With sinus arrest,
the PP intervals are irregular with long pauses (which are not
multiples of the basic sinus interval) intervening (Fig. 4*B*). Sinoatrial block is suspected when the intervening pauses between
P waves are simple multiples of each other. Sinoatrial block may
be a manifestation of digitalis intoxication or electrolytic disturbance,[43, 50] which should be corrected if this is the case. Sinoatrial block or even periods of sinus arrest are not uncom-
monly seen during laryngoscopy for tracheal intubation in the
absence of effective vagal blockade. Distinction between bradycardia caused by sinoatrial block or sinus arrest, and sinus arrhythmia is usually not a problem (Fig. 5). Sinus arrhythmia is
diagnosed when the intervals between P waves vary by more
than 0.12 seconds.[43] It is most often characterized by an increase in heart rate during inspiration and a decrease following
exhalation (phasic sinus arrhythmia). In older individuals, however, the variation in heart rate may be unrelated to respiration
(nonphasic sinus arrhythmia). At times the irregularity of pulse
beats or heart sounds may be so striking that sinus arrhythmia
may resemble atrial fibrillation. The true cause of the irregularity
becomes apparent when its relation to respiration is determined
or the ECG reveals the nature of the irregularity. Sinus arrhythmia is a normal finding in children and young adults, is usually
absent in middle age, and may reappear with advancing age.[43]

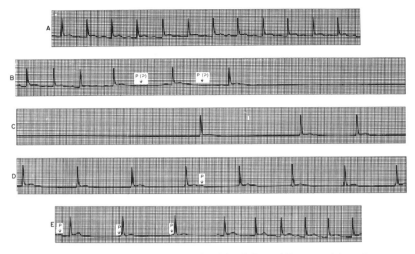

Figure 4. Sinus arrest and sinoatrial block in a 17-year-old male patient with Grave's disease who is undergoing subtotal thyroidectomy. Preoperatively, the patient was in first-degree AV block. He had been receiving methylthiouracil and propranolol (20 mg p.o., q.i.d.) preoperatively. A, Sinus rhythm with first-degree AV block (PR = 0.22 seconds) prior to the induction of anesthesia (electrocardiographic lead II). The induction consisted of Innovar[R] and thiopental I.V., and nitrous oxide-oxygen. Succinylcholine was used for intubation. B, C, D, and E, Continuous recording (electrocardiographic lead II) of heart rhythm during laryngoscopy for the topical application of 160 mg of 4 percent lidocaine to the tracheal mucosa. The absent P waves in B, before complete sinus arrest, are probably due to sinoatrial block. An approximate 10-second period of sinus arrest (B and C) is followed by a slow, junctional escape rhythm (C and D). A single P wave is noted in D. This and the first three P waves in E fail to capture the ventricles (AV dissociation). The fourth and succeeding P waves capture the ventricles, but with long PR intervals (0.20 to 0.22 seconds).

Sinus arrhythmia in older persons, however, may be a sign of disordered sinus function.

Neither sinoatrial block, short periods of sinus arrest, nor sinus arrhythmia require specific treatment unless they are symptomatic or impair circulatory function. Small doses of atropine given intravenously are effective in treating these disturbances. In the nontoxic digitalized patient, persistent sinoatrial

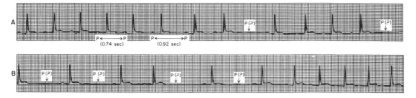

Figure 5. Nonphasic sinus arrhythmia, sinoatrial block, and first-degree AV block in the patient in Figure 4. This arrhythmia was noted after the administration of ephedrine (10 mg I.V.) during endotracheal intubation. Note the variation in PP intervals (0.74 to 0.92 msec) during sinus arrhythmia, and the absence of P waves during sinoatrial block. The recordings in A and B are contiguous.

block demands caution in administering additional digitalis for its inotropic effect, unless a ventricular pacemaker is present.[50]

Sinus bradycardia, sinus arrest, sinoatrial block, or sinus arrhythmia (especially the nonphasic variety) may occur on a chronic basis as a manifestation of the sick sinus syndrome.[43, 50-53] In patients with the sick sinus syndrome, episodes of sinus arrest or sinoatrial block may not be associated with drug therapy and may be followed by the development of escape rhythms. The slow heart rate allows escape of multiple potential ectopic pacemaker sites, promotes a wide temporal dispersion of repolarization in the heart, and sets up the circumstances that promote a wide variety of re-entrant arrhythmias.[50] Indeed, bradycardia predisposes the patient to tachycardia, and supraventricular or ventricular tachyarrhythmias may complicate the picture in more than half the patients with the sick sinus syndrome.[52] The association of bradycardia with tachyarrhythmias is referred to as the brady-tachy syndrome.[54] Disturbances of AV conduction are frequently associated with the sick sinus syndrome.[50] Since the treatment of the supraventricular arrhythmias with drugs such as quinidine may aggravate the AV conduction block, most patients with the sick sinus syndrome are managed with pacemakers.[50, 52, 53] Patients with the sick sinus syndrome without a pacemaker are at increased risk of developing bradyarrhythmias during the perioperative period. Pacemakers do not prevent the development of tachyarrhythmias, but may be used to treat them by overdrive suppression, that is, the heart is driven at a rate faster than that of the ectopic pacemaker, thereby suppressing it and terminating the tachycardia.

AV junctional and *idioventricular rhythm* are causes of brady-cardia that may be related to drugs or to sinus node dysfunction. When digitalis excess is a cause, this should be treated prior to surgery by withholding further digitalis. Hypokalemia or hypo-magnesemia in patients receiving digitalis may also be respon-sible for these rhythm disturbances and should be corrected. When surgery is urgent and these rhythm disturbances are pres-ent, temporary electronic pacing is indicated because of the real danger of further downward migration of the pacemaker or asystole upon exposure to anesthetics. It would be dangerous under such circumstances to rely totally on pharmacologic means to increase the automaticity of subsidiary pacemaker foci. The appearance of junctional rhythm during anesthesia is not uncommon (Figs. 5 and 6). If this occurs during deep levels of anesthesia, it should be corrected by reducing the concentra-tion of anesthetic agent, or by substituting drugs with a less de-pressant effect on sinus function.

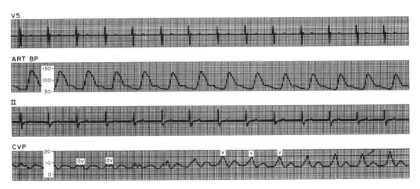

Figure 6. Recordings of the electrocardiographic leads V₅ and II, and the arterial (Art) and central venous pressure (CVP) in a 72-year-old male undergoing coronary bypass surgery. The patient is in sinus rhythm on the left side of the tracings, but progresses to midjunctional rhythm on the right side. Note the concomitant fall in arterial blood pressure and development of large v waves in the CVP. A sudden drop in arterial pressure or the development of large v waves in the CVP are suggestive of downward migration of the pacemaker in the absence of immediately recognizable changes in the ECG. The heart sounds softened and became less audible with the development of the arrhythmia.

ANESTHESIA AND THE PATIENT WITH HEART DISEASE

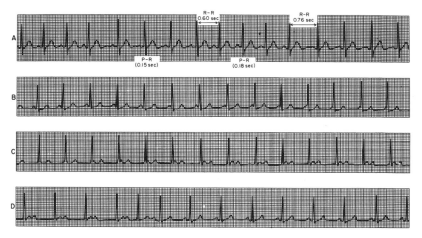

Figure 7. Wandering atrial pacemaker (A) and isorhythmic AV dissociation (B and D). A, Tracing (electrocardiographic lead II) from a 67-year-old diabetic female undergoing a right lumbar sympathectomy. The anesthetic was N$_2$O-O$_2$-halothane. Note that the P waves vary in configuration and the PR intervals range from 0.15 to 0.18 seconds. The RR intervals vary between 0.60 and 0.76 seconds. B, C, and D, Progression of P waves in and out of the QRS complex without a change in their configuration is a feature of isorhythmic AV dissociation. Tracings B and C were made later in the procedure. As the anesthetic was lightened near the end of the procedure, the arrhythmia disappeared with return to sinus rhythm (D).

Wandering atrial pacemaker and *isorhythmic AV dissociation* (Fig. 7) are arrhythmias commonly seen during anesthesia. Wandering atrial pacemaker is diagnosed when the P waves vary in morphology but the QRS complexes are definitely supraventricular in origin, that is, they have a normal appearance. The PR intervals may also vary in wandering atrial pacemaker. Isorhythmic AV dissociation means that the atria and ventricles beat independently of each other. It is distinguished from complete AV block by the "supraventricular" appearance of the QRS complexes and the constant relationship (PR or RP interval) between P waves and QRS complexes. Both these rhythm disturbances may be a cause of bradycardia, associated with significant hypotension. They are frequently seen in patients deeply anesthetized with potent inhalation agents such as halothane or enflurane, particularly when these drugs are used as the sole anesthetic agent. Almost invariably, sinus rhythm can be restored by lightening the level of anesthesia. If the bradycardia and hypotension must be reversed urgently, a vasopressor with mixed alpha and beta activity (e.g., ephedrine or mephentermine) is preferred to atropine, which might be a cause of far more serious arrhythmias.[48]

Tachyarrhythmias

Tachycardia is manifest by a heart rate greater than 100 beats per minute in adults; greater than 120 beats per minute in children; and greater than 140 beats per minute in infants.[43] Tachycardias may be of sinus, atrial, AV junctional, or ventricular origin and may be nonparoxysmal or paroxysmal. Paroxysmal tachycardias are characterized by their abrupt onset, usually within one cardiac cycle, and sudden termination. With sinus tachycardia, the onset and termination are more gradual. Nonparoxysmal tachycardia implies that the rhythm disturbance is established, and includes atrial flutter or fibrillation, ventricular tachycardia, and ventricular fibrillation.

Tachycardias are dangerous to the extent that they interfere with normal cardiac output and favorable relationship between myocardial oxygen supply and demand. As a group, tachyarrhythmias are the most serious arrhythmias likely to be encountered in the perioperative environment. Their occurrence demands immediate attention. Functionally, the lower the pacemaker responsible for the tachycardia, the more likely the tachycardia is to be hemodynamically significant. Ventricular tachycardia is more serious than supraventricular tachycardia. It is more likely to signify elevation of the left ventricular end-diastolic pressure and a marked fall in the cardiac output. This will cause hypotension, inadequate perfusion of vital organs, pulmonary edema, and cardiorespiratory arrest. An untreated ventricular tachycardia will progress to ventricular fibrillation, the most serious arrhythmia, since effective cardiac output ceases with this arrhythmia.

Sinus tachycardia is the most common rhythm disturbance in the perioperative setting. The usual causes are a decrease in effective blood volume, fever, pain, hypoxia, hypercarbia, acidosis, and drugs that stimulate the sympathetic or block the parasympathetic components of the autonomic nervous system. There is no specific therapy for sinus tachycardia other than removal of the precipitating cause, except in patients with coronary artery disease, in whom propranolol (1.0 to 3.0 mg I.V. in divided doses) is indicated if signs or symptoms of ischemia are present. It is sometimes difficult to distinguish sinus tachycardia with a rate above 150 beats per minute from a paroxysmal supraventricular tachycardia. Several distinguishing features of these two types of arrhythmias may be helpful. With sinus tachycardia, the onset is more gradual, the cause for the tachycardia (e.g., fever, blood loss, or drugs) is more apparent, and some small amount of variation in the heart rate is usually seen with repeated observations.[43] With paroxysmal supraventricular tachycardia, the onset is abrupt, there is no obvious reason for the tachycardia, and the heart rate is constant over a period of time.[43] Other distinguishing features between sinus tachycardia and paroxysmal supraventricular tachycardia include responses to carotid sinus pressure or cholinergic interventions (e.g., edrophonium, neostigmine), and P wave characteristics (information follows).

Paroxysmal supraventricular tachycardias may be due to enhanced irritability in atrial ectopic focus, re-entry within the atria or AV junctional tissues, or the Wolff-Parkinson-White syndrome.[43, 50] The atrial rate usually ranges from 140 to 220 beats per minute, and there is usually 1:1 AV conduction response.[50] The P waves may be indiscernible or of abnormal appearance, as opposed to the normal P waves seen in sinus tachycardia. The QRS complexes are normal in appearance unless there is associated aberrant ventricular conduction. In the absence of discernible P waves and the presence of aberrant ventricular conduction, paroxysmal supraventricular tachycardia may be extremely difficult to distinguish from ventricular tachycardia. Paroxysmal supraventricular tachycardias may be abruptly converted to normal (slow) sinus rhythm by application of carotid sinus pressure, or intravenous administration of edrophonium (10 mg) or neostigmine (1.0 mg). These interventions virtually never affect ventricular tachycardia. AV flutter or fibrillation may respond to carotid sinus massage by an increase in the degree of AV block and temporary slowing of the ventricular rate lasting as long as carotid sinus pressure is applied. In sinus tachycardia there may be a modest slowing (10 to 20 beats per minute) in the sinus rate, which returns to its previous level when the carotid sinus pressure is released.

Carotid sinus pressure is applied just above the bifurcation of the common carotid artery, which is approximately at the level of the superior border of the larynx. It should be applied on one side only, and never for more than 5 seconds at a time. Carotid sinus pressure may be more effective when used in combination with positive airway pressure, the Valsalva maneuver, a vasopressor such as methoxamine (5 to 10 mg) or phenylephrine (0.5 to 1.0 mg), or a cholinesterase inhibitor (10 mg edrophonium, or 1.0 mg neostigmine). Frequently, a paroxysmal supraventricular tachycardia may be terminated by the use of edrophonium or neostigmine alone. Carotid sinus pressure should not be used in elderly patients, in those with carotid bruits, or in patients with a high degree of AV block. Vasopressors are potentially dangerous in patients with coronary artery disease, since failure to restore sinus rhythm could result in both tachycardia and hypertension. Only vasopressors with alpha-adrenergic activity (e.g., methoxamine, phenylephrine) should be used, and only in an amount necessary to achieve a blood pressure of 140 to 160 torr systolic. Because of the potential dangers associated with the use of carotid sinus pressure and vasopressors, it is frequently preferable to use anticholinesterase therapy alone or in combination with positive airway pressure in anesthetized patients. When a paroxysmal supraventricular tachycardia fails to respond to these measures, additional therapy includes drugs, such as digitalis or propranolol to slow the ventricular rate, or even electrical conversion. Temporary rapid atrial pacing may be effective in terminating the arrhythmia (through overdrive suppression) or converting it to atrial fibrillation, in which case digitalis can be used to slow the ventricular response.[55]

Nonparoxysmal supraventricular tachycardias other than atrial flutter or fibrillation include atrial tachycardia with block and multifocal atrial tachycardia with or without block.[43] An example of the latter type of arrhythmia, commonly referred to as chaotic atrial mechanism, is seen in Figure 3B. These arrhythmias are most commonly related to chronic pulmonary disease,[50] digitalis intoxication,[56] diabetes mellitus,[50] or end-stage heart disease.[57] The usual atrial rate is somewhere between 140 and 200 beats per minute.[50] The P waves appear different from those of sinus origin, but the PR intervals are not as short as in a high junctional tachycardia. There is often variation in the PP intervals, and the electrocardiographic baseline is isoelectric between P waves, in contrast to atrial flutter or fibrillation.[50] AV block in association with atrial tachycardia is often of the

Wenckenbach (Mobitz I) type, with highly variable AV conduction ratios.[50] Unless caused by treatable factors, such as electrolyte imbalances or digitalis excess, these arrhythmias may be difficult to suppress. Electrical conversion is usually not effective, since the rhythm disturbance frequently recurs.[58] If the arrhythmia is related to digitalis excess, the threshold for ventricular fibrillation is lowered, making cardioversion more risky.[58] Phenytoin (I.V.) may be effective for these arrhythmias when caused by digitalis excess.[59] Quinidine and procainamide may be used in these patients to slow the atrial rate,[50] but both these drugs when given parenterally during general anesthesia have the potential for additive myocardial depression and vasodilation.[44]

Atrial flutter or fibrillation may be associated with rheumatic valvular disease, coronary artery disease, hypertension, or hypermetabolic states and is frequently seen in patients during or following major pulmonary or cardiovascular procedures. Atrial flutter is recognized by the characteristic rhythmic oscillations (240 to 400 per minute)[50] of the baseline with no isoelectric periods between flutter waves (Fig. 8). There is usually a 2:1

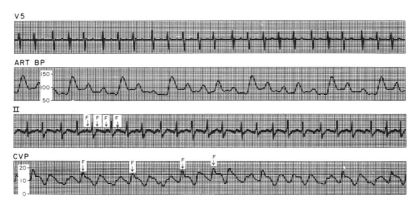

Figure 8. Atrial flutter that developed at the time of atrial cannulization in patient in Figure 6. Flutter waves (F) are apparent in lead II. There is 2:1 AV block with the ventricular rate approximately 150 beats per minute. Note the trigeminal pattern of the arterial pulse contour (pulsus alternans), and the superposition of flutter (F) waves on the v waves in the CVP (compare with Figure 6). Changes in the appearance of the central venous pressure waveform can be extremely helpful in the clinical detection and diagnosis of disturbances in cardiac rhythm.

AV conduction block, and the ventricular rate will vary between 120 and 200 beats per minute.[50] The flutter waves may be more easily recognized following the application of carotid sinus pressure or administration of edrophonium to slow the ventricular rate. Atrial fibrillation is characterized by irregular oscillations (400 to 600 per minute) of the electrocardiographic baseline.[50] The ventricular rate in untreated atrial fibrillation is highly irregular and may range from 100 to 200 beats per minute.[50] Both atrial flutter and fibrillation are treated with digitalis to slow the ventricular response. If the patient is in overt heart failure or shows signs of coronary ischemia and requires immediate therapy, direct cardioversion is indicated. In the presence of digitalis, DC cardioversion should only be attempted with much decreased voltage. Phenytoin, which increases the ventricular fibrillation threshold, may be administered prior to counter shock in digitalized patients.[50, 58, 60] Patients with recurrent episodes of atrial fibrillation or flutter are continued on digitalis. Procainamide or quinidine may be used in such patients in an attempt to maintain sinus rhythm.[59]

The recognition and management of ventricular tachycardia or fibrillation are well established and will not be discussed here. When ventricular tachycardia results from digitalis intoxication, however, DC counter shock should be used only after lidocaine or other drug therapy has been unsuccessful, or if the blood pressure has fallen dramatically. In the absence of hyperkalemia, potassium chloride may be effective in controlling arrhythmias caused by digitalis. Intravenous propranolol (up to a total dose of 3 mg) or phenytoin may also be effective.[43]

AV Conduction Block

The phrase AV conduction block indicates that there is some impairment in the conduction of electrical impulses from the atria to the ventricles. In first-degree AV block, there is a delay in conduction of impulses to the ventricles. The PR interval is longer than 0.20 seconds in adults with heart rates between 70 and 90 beats per minute.[43] The normal AV conduction time is affected by heart rate. The normal upper limits for the PR interval in an adult are 0.21 seconds for a heart rate of 60 beats per minute, and 0.19 seconds for a heart rate of 90 beats per minute.[43] AV conduction time is less in infants and children, so that in a child of 5 years, the normal upper limit is 0.16 seconds when the heart rate is 100 beats per minute.[43] With very rapid heart rates, for example, during a supraventricular tachycardia or electrical pacing of the atria, it is possible to observe degrees of AV block when the rate exceeds the relative refractory period of the AV node. This is a physiologic and protective response.

Second-degree AV block exists when some, but not all, atrial impulses are conducted to the ventricles. Three types are recognized. In Mobitz Type I (Wenckebach) block, the PR interval progressively lengthens before the dropped ventricular beat. In Mobitz Type II, although the PR interval remains constant, some ventricular beats are dropped. When three or more atrial impulses in succession are blocked, this is called advanced second-degree block. The ratio between atrial and ventricular complexes is usually specified (e.g., 7:8, 6:5, or 4:3 block). With third-degree or complete AV block, no atrial beats result in ventricular capture. Complete AV block is distinguished from AV dissociation by interference.[43] The latter phrase implies that the atrial impulses do not capture the ventricles because they fall within the AV nodal refractory period, which may be prolonged by drugs or disease. Isorhythmic dissociation (see Fig. 7) is an example of AV dissociation by interference.

Since first-degree AV block by itself is rarely symptomatic or associated with a significant reduction in cardiac output, it usually does not require treatment. It can be considered a therapeutic effect of digitalis.[50] When associated with sinus bradycardia, it may become symptomatic or hemodynamically significant. Since atropine is effective in treating this condition, it is usually all that is required.

Mobitz Type I block is also considered a relatively benign form of rhythm disturbance, since the ventricular rate is usually adequate to support perfusion of vital organs. While the conduction defect responsible for this type of block may be anywhere within the AV conducting system, it is usually within the AV node.[61] Atropine, by removing vagal influences, will reverse the block or establish a higher atrial to ventricular conduction ratio. Mobitz Type I block may be due to digitalis excess. The use of an artificial pacemaker is not indicated for surgical procedures performed on patients with Mobitz Type I block, unless the block is symptomatic or associated with significant reductions in cardiac output, and the block cannot be reversed by drug administration. While experimental evidence indicates that anesthetics prolong AV conduction in a dose-related manner,[62-64] there is no evidence that patients with first-degree or Mobitz Type I block are likely to develop more advanced degrees of block during anesthesia and surgery. This may be due to the enhanced sympathetic tone induced by the stress of surgery or to the lighter levels of anesthesia generally chosen for these patients.

Mobitz Type II block is a more serious form of block, since it is frequently associated with disease of the His-Purkinje tissues.[61] In patients with myocardial infarction, the onset of this type of block can be abrupt, and it may progress to complete AV block with unpredictable rapidity.[65] When Mobitz II block progresses to complete AV block, the escape ventricular rhythms that develop are slow (less than 50 beats per minute) and manifest widened, bizarre QRS complexes.[50] Since drug treatment is not reliable in patients with Mobitz Type II block, permanent ventricular pacing is indicated.[50] These same considerations apply to advanced second-degree block.

Permanent ventricular pacing is indicated for all patients with complete AV block except those with the congenital form.[43] In patients with congenital complete heart block, the intrinsic pacemaker is usually located within the AV junction or His's bundle, and the QRS complex is of normal duration.[66] In one group of patients with this problem, the ventricular rates varied between 45 and 85 beats per minute.[67] With acquired complete block, the QRS complexes are more widened and bizarre in appearance, and the ventricular rates are 50 beats per minute or below. Even though patients with acquired complete block may be asymptomatic, they often feel better after the insertion of an artificial pacemaker to increase the ventricular rate.[68] A ventricular pacemaker is absolutely indicated prior to anesthesia and surgery in all patients with acquired complete heart block. In congenital complete heart block the indication for artificial pacing is determined by the symptoms and the range of ventricular rates in response to exercise.

Block of conduction may also occur within the bundle branches or principal divisions (anterior and posterior fascicles) of the left bundle branch. Left anterior hemiblock is diagnosed when the QRS complex is of normal duration and its axis is between -40 and -80 degrees, although some clinicians would make the diagnosis when the QRS axis was more negative than

−30 degrees in the absence of an inferior infarction.[43] Left posterior hemiblock is suspected when the QRS complex is not prolonged and the axis between +80 and +120 degrees.[61] Left anterior hemiblock is commonly found in association with right bundle branch block.[61] Left posterior hemiblock alone is rare; when it is seen, it is usually in patients with right bundle branch block.[61]

The question of whether or not an electronic pacemaker is indicated for patients with bifascicular block plagues anesthesiologists, cardiologists, and surgeons, alike. The problem is whether the block will progress to complete AV block during surgery or during anesthesia because of drugs. There is insufficient data to support either position. Several recent studies indicate that patients with asymptomatic right bundle branch block do not develop complete AV block during general anesthesia and surgery,[70-72] and ventricular pacing is not indicated for this particular group of patients. However, we feel it is indicated in symptomatic patients with bifascicular block (right bundle branch plus either anterior or posterior hemiblock), or when bifascicular block occurs in association with second-degree AV block. Isolated right bundle branch block does not require treatment. Left bundle branch block that is symptomatic or associated with second-degree AV block is an indication for therapy with an electronic pacemaker.

SUMMARY

Cardiac arrhythmias are extremely common in the perioperative setting. They only require treatment when they (1) interfere significantly with normal tissue perfusion; (2) adversely affect the normal balance between myocardial oxygen supply and demand; or (3) predispose the patient to ventricular tachycardia or fibrillation. Usually, the treatment is simple: correct the underlying cause or causes. In some instances, either the cause will not be apparent or time will not permit adequate identification of the precipitating events. In these instances, drug treatment or electrical therapy is indicated. The classification of arrhythmias and the actions, indications, dosages and routes, and major side effects of the drugs commonly used in their treatment are summarized in Tables 1 through 3. The indications for electrical therapy, including pacemakers and cardioversion, were discussed in the sections dealing with bradyarrhythmias, tachyarrhythmias, and AV conduction block.

ACKNOWLEDGMENTS

The author wishes to express his sincere appreciation to his following colleagues, whose suggestions were helpful in the preparation of this chapter: Dr. Betty J. Bamforth, Dr. Brian H. Hoff, and Dr. W. Stuart Sykes.

REFERENCES

1. Hoffman, B. F., and Cranefield, P. F.: *Electrophysiology of the Heart.* McGraw-Hill, New York, 1960.
2. DeMello, W. C.(ed.): *Electrical Phenomena in the Heart.* Academic Press, New York, 1972.
3. Noble, D.: *The Initiation of the Heart Beat.* Clarendon Press, Oxford, England, 1975.
4. Cranefield, P. F.: *The Conduction of the Cardiac Impulse.* Futura Publishing Company, Mount Kisco, New York, 1975.
5. Narula, O. S.: *His Bundle Electrocardiography and Clinical Electrophysiology.* F.A. Davis Company, Philadelphia, 1975.
6. Akhtar, M., and Damato, A. N.: *Clinical uses of His-bundle electrocardiography. Part 1.* Am. Heart J. 91:520, 1976.
7. Akhtar, M., Damato, A. N., and Caracta, A. R.: *Clinical uses of His-bundle electrocardiography. Part 2.* Am. Heart J. 91:660, 1976.
8. Akhtar, M., Damato, A. N., Lau, S. H., et al.: *Clinical uses of His-bundle electrocardiography. Part 3.* Am. Heart J. 91:805, 1976.
9. Cranefield, P. F., Wit, A. L., and Hoffman, B. F.: *Genesis of cardiac arrhythmias.* Circulation 47:190, 1973.
10. Ferrier, G. R.: *Digitalis arrhythmias: role of oscillatory afterpotentials.* Prog. Cardiovasc. Dis. 19:459, 1977.
11. Cranefield, P. F.: *Action potentials, after potentials and arrhythmias.* Circ. Res. 41:415, 1977.
12. Tsein, R. W., and Carpenter, D. O.: *Ionic mechanisms of pacemaker activity in cardiac Purkinje fibers.* Fed. Proc. 37:2127, 1978.
13. Moe, G.K.: *Evidence for re-entry as a mechanism of cardiac arrhythmias.* Rev. Physiol. Biochem. Pharmacol. 72:55, 1975.
14. Katz, R. L.: *Neural factors affecting cardiac arrhythmias induced by halopropane.* J. Pharmacol. Exp. Ther. 152:88, 1966.
15. Price, H. L., Lurie, A. A., Jones, R. E., et al.: *Cyclopropane anesthesia. I. Cardiac rate and rhythm during steady levels of cyclopropane anesthesia at normal and elevated end-expiratory carbon dioxide tensions.* Anesthesiology 19:457, 1958.

16. Price, H. L., Lurie, A. A., Jones, R. E. et al.: *Cyclopropane anesthesia. II. Epinephrine and norepinephrine in initiation of ventricular arrhythmias by carbon dioxide inhalation.* Anesthesiology 19:619, 1958.
17. Black, G. W., Linde, H. W., Dripps, R. D. et al.: *Circulatory changes accompanying respiratory acidosis during halothane (Fluothane) anaesthesia in man.* Br. J. Anaesth. 31:238, 1959.
18. Edwards, R., Winnie, A. P., and Ramamurphy, S.: *Acute hypocapneic hypokalemia: an iatrogenic anesthetic complication.* Anesth. Analg. (Cleve.) 56:786, 1977.
19. Reynolds, A. K., Chiz, J. F., and Pasquet, A. F.: *Halothane and methoxyflurane—a comparison of their effects on cardiac pacemaker fibers.* Anesthesiology 33:602, 1970.
20. Smith, N. T., Calverley, R. K., Jones, C. W., et al.: *The hemodynamic impact of atrial arrhythmias during enflurane anesthesia in man.* Abstracts of Scientific Papers, American Society of Anesthesiologists Annual Meeting, New Orleans, 1977, pp. 99–100.
21. Smith, N. T.: Personal communication, 1978.
22. Katz, R. L., and Epstein, R. A.: *The interaction of anesthetic agents and adrenergic drugs to produce cardiac arrhythmias.* Anesthesiology 29:763, 1968.
23. Johnston, R. R., Eger, E. I., and Wilson, C.: *A comparative interaction of epinephrine with enflurane, isoflurane, and halothane in man.* Anesth. Analg. (Cleve.) 56:378, 1977.
24. Katz, R. L., and Bigger, J. T., Jr.: *Cardiac arrhythmias during anesthesia and operation.* Anesthesiology 33:192, 1970.
25. Prys-Roberts, C., Foëx, P., Biro, G. P., et al.: *Studies of anaesthesia in relation to hypertension. V. Adrenergic beta-receptor blockade.* Br. J. Anaesth. 45:671, 1973.
26. Schoenstadt, D. A., and Whitcher, C. E.: *Observations on the mechanism of succinylcholine-induced cardiac arrhythmias.* Anesthesiology 24:358, 1963.
27. Lowenstein, E.: *Succinylcholine administration in the burned patient.* Anesthesiology 27:494, 1966.
28. Tolmie, J. D., Joyce, T. H., and Mitchell, G. D.: *Succinylcholine: danger in the burned patient.* Anesthesiology 28:467, 1967.
29. Gronert, G. A., Dotin, L. A., Ritchey, C. R., et al.: *Succinylcholine-induced hyperkalemia in burned patients—II.* Anesth. Analg. (Cleve.) 48:958, 1969.
30. Birch, A. A., Mitchell, G. D., Playford, G. A., et al.: *Changes in serum potassium response to succinylcholine following trauma.* J.A.M.A. 210:490, 1969.
31. Kopriva, C., Ratliff, J., Fletcher, J. R., et al.: *Serum potassium changes after succinylcholine in patients with acute massive muscle trauma.* Anesthesiology 34:246, 1971.

32. Mazze, R. E., Escue, H. M., and Houston, J. B.: *Hyperkalemia and cardiovascular collapse following administration of succinylcholine to the traumatized patient.* Anesthesiology 31:540, 1969.
33. Cooperman, L. H.: *Succinylcholine-induced hyperkalemia in neuromuscular disease.* J.A.M.A. 213:1867, 1970.
34. Tobey, R. E.: *Paraplegia, succinylcholine, and cardiac arrest.* Anesthesiology 32:359, 1970.
35. Genever, E. E.: *Suxamethonium-induced cardiac arrest in unsuspected pseudohypertrophic muscular dystrophy.* Br. J. Anaesth. 43:984, 1971.
36. Smith, R. B., and Grenvik, A.: *Cardiac arrest following succinylcholine in patients with central nervous system injuries.* Anesthesiology 33:558, 1970.
37. Tobey, R. E., Jacobsen, P. M., Kahle, C. T., et al.: *The serum potassium response to muscle relaxants in neural injury.* Anesthesiology 37:332, 1972.
38. John, D. A., Tobey, R. E., Homer, L. D., et al.: *Onset of succinylcholine-induced hyperkalemia following denervation.* Anesthesiology 45:294, 1976.
39. Kohlschütter, B., Baur, H., and Roth, F.: *Suxamethonium-induced hyperkalemia in patients with severe intra-abdominal infections.* Br. J. Anaesth. 48:557, 1976.
40. Dowdy, E. G., and Fabian, L. W.: *Ventricular arrhythmias induced by succinylcholine in digitalized patients.* Anesth. Analg. (Cleve.) 42:501, 1963.
41. Dowdy, E. G., Duggar, P. N., and Fabian, L. W.: *Effect of neuromuscular blocking agents on isolated digitalized mammalian hearts.* Anesth. Analg. (Cleve.) 44:608, 1965.
42. Schwartz, H.: "Oculocardiac reflex: Is prophylaxis necessary?" In Mark, L. C., and Ngai, S. H. (eds): *Highlights of Clinical Anesthesiology.* Harper & Row, New York, 1971, pp. 111–114.
43. Fowler, N. O.: *Cardiac Diagnosis and Treatment,* ed. 2. Harper & Row, New York, 1976, pp. 889–978.
44. Moe, G. K., and Abildskov, J. A.: "Antiarrhythmic Drugs." In Goodman, L. S., and Gilman, A.(eds.): *The Pharmacological Basis of Therapeutics,* ed. 5. MacMillan, New York, 1975, pp. 683–704.
45. Lang, T. W., Bernstein, H., Barbieri, F. F., et al.: *The use of diphenylhydantoin for the treatment of digitalis toxicity.* Arch. Intern. Med. 116:573, 1965.
46. Bigger, J. T., Jr., Schmidt, D. H., and Kutt, H.: *Relationship between plasma level of diphenylhydantoin sodium and its cardiac antiarrhythmic effects.* Circulation 38:363, 1968.
47. Das, G., Talmers, F. N., and Weissler, A. M.: *New observations on the effects of atropine on the sinoatrial and atrioventricular nodes in man.* Am. J. Cardiol. 36:281, 1975.

48. Jones, R. E., Deutsch, S., and Turndorf, H.: *Effects of atropine on cardiac rhythm in conscious and anesthetized man.* Anesthesiology 22:67, 1961.
49. Greenblatt, D. J., and Shader, R. I.: *Anticholinergics.* N. Engl. J. Med. 288:1215, 1973.
50. Warner, H.: *Therapy of common arrhythmias.* Med. Clin. North Am. 58:995, 1974.
51. Ferrer, M. I.: *The Sick Sinus Syndrome.* Futura Publishing Co., Inc. Mt. Kisco, New York, 1974.
52. Bower, P. J.: *Sick sinus syndrome.* Arch. Intern. Med. 138:133, 1978.
53. Scarpa, W. J.: *The sick sinus syndrome.* Am. Heart J. 92:648, 1976.
54. Moss, A. J., and Davis, R. J.: *Brady-tachy syndrome.* Prog. Cardiovasc. Dis. 16:439, 1974.
55. Pittman, D. E., Makar, J.S., Kooros, K. S., et al.: *Rapid atrial stimulation: successful method of conversion of atrial flutter and atrial tachycardia.* Am. J. Cardiol. 32:700, 1973.
56. Chung, E. K.: *Digitalis-induced cardiac arrhythmias.* Am. Heart J. 79:845, 1970.
57. Chung, E. K.: *Appraisal of multifocal atrial tachycardia.* Br. Heart J. 33:500, 1971.
58. Szekely, P., Wynne, N. A., Pearson, D. T., et al.: *Direct current shock and digitalis, a clinical and experimental study.* Br. Heart J. 31:91, 1969.
59. Bigger, J. T.: *Arrhythmias and antiarrhythmic drugs.* Adv. Intern. Med. 18:158, 1972.
60. Helfant, R. H., Scherlag, B. J., and Damato, A. N.: *Diphenylhydantoin prevention of arrhythmias in the digitalis-sensitized dog after direct current cardioversion.* Circulation 37:424, 1968.
61. Kastor, J. A.: *Atrioventricular block (first of two parts).* N. Engl. J. Med. 292:462, 1975.
62. Atlee, J. L., and Rusy, B. F.: *Halothane depression of A-V conduction studied by electrograms of the bundle of His in dogs.* Anesthesiology 36:112, 1972.
63. Atlee, J. L., Homer, L. D., and Tobey, R. E.: *Diphenylhydantoin and lidocaine modification of A-V conduction in halothane-anesthetized dogs.* Anesthesiology 43:49, 1975.
64. Atlee, J. L., and Rusy, B. F.: *Atrioventricular conduction times and atrioventricular nodal conductivity during enflurane anesthesia in dogs.* Anesthesiology 47:498, 1977.
65. Stock, R. J., and Macken, D. L.: *Observations on heart block during continuous electrocardiographic monitoring in acute myocardial infarction.* Circulation 38:993, 1968.
66. Scarpelli, E. M., and Rudolph, A. M.: *The hemodynamics of congenital heart block.* Prog. Cardiovasc. Dis. 6:327, 1964.
67. Paul, M. H., Rudolph, A. M., and Nadas, A. S.: *Congenital complete*

atrioventricular block: problems of clinical assessment. Circulation 18:183, 1958.
68. Kastor, J. A.: *Atrioventricular block (second of two parts).* N. Engl. J. Med. 292:572, 1975.
69. Rosenbaum, B., Elizari, M. V., and Lazzari, J. O.: *The Hemiblocks.* Tampa Tracings, Oldsmar, Florida, 1970.
70. Venkataraman, K., Madias, J. E., Hood, W. B., Jr.: *Indications for prophylactic preoperative insertion of pacemakers in patients with right bundle branch block and left anterior hemiblock.* Chest 68:501, 1975.
71. Rooney, S.M., Goldimer, P. L., and Muss, E.: *Relationship of right bundle branch block and marked left axis deviation to complete heart block during general anesthesia.* Anesthesiology 44:64, 1976.
72. Pastore, J. O., Yurchak, P. M., Janis, K. M., et al.: *The risk of advanced heart block in surgical patients with right bundle branch block and left axis deviation.* Circulation 57:677, 1978.

POSTOPERATIVE CARE OF THE PATIENT WITH HEART DISEASE

Joseph C. Gabel, M.D., and
Alan S. Tonnesen, M.D.

Proper and safe management of the cardiac patient scheduled for surgery begins in the preoperative phase with careful assessment so that an anesthetic game-plan can be devised. Obviously, intraoperative management always holds the primary focus for the anesthesiologist. Yet, as far as cardiac mortality and morbidity are concerned, the postoperative phase is the most crucial. Myocardial infarction or reinfarction is more prone to occur within the first 72 hours postoperatively than it is intraoperatively. Drs. Gabel and Tonnesen discuss the important aspect of immediate postoperative care for the cardiac patient.

Burnell R. Brown, Jr.

Postoperative care, a continuation and reflection of the preoperative and operative management, may be defined as beginning when the last stitch is placed in the patient's skin. An interim period then follows when the patient is transferred from the operating table to his bed and transported to the recovery room. This interim period may involve considerable time and is a period when the vigilance and precision of observation that mark the operative period are often relaxed, and care may be actually quite cursory. This chapter will be principally concerned with the next 48 to 72 hours, the immediate postoperative period. The majority of acute complications occur during this period and skillful management can make the difference between life and death.

Discussion of this period can be divided into basic principles, accurate assessment of the cardiovascular state, and the prevention and treatment of complications. The main theme of this chapter is that *there is no substitute for continuous and accurate assessment* of the patient's condition. Deterioration of the cardiopulmonary system is usually insidious and becomes more difficult (if not impossible) to reverse when not quickly detected and corrected. The intensity of assessment necessary is judged from the preoperative evaluation, the operative procedure, and the intraoperative course. A simple regimen is sufficient for straightforward cases, but a comprehensive regimen is indicated for the more complicated and difficult cases. The goal of each scheme of management is to obtain adequate data to determine, before a crisis develops, which of the patient's systems, if any, is deteriorating and what is the urgency of therapeutic intervention. It should be emphasized that simple measures can be corrective if deterioration is diagnosed early enough.

BASIC PRINCIPLES

Specific requirements of staffing of nurses need to be determined by local factors, such as the types of surgical procedures performed and the availability of other postoperative care areas. The important nursing concept is the identity of the *recovery room as an intensive care area.* If patients with serious underlying cardiac disease are to successfully recover from major operative procedures, the postoperative care must be directed toward the care of the acutely ill. The concept of a recovery room as only a place to recover from anesthesia is outmoded and unacceptable. The essence of this identity lies not in the level of care given to the majority of patients, but rather the care available to those whose status requires it.

The emphasis on the care of the acutely ill is not meant to minimize the importance of comfortable and restful accommodations; it is meant to establish the necessity of a nursing orientation that is physiologically based in the cardiovascular, respiratory, and renal systems. It may well be said that far more medical judgment, on the part of both the anesthetists and nurses, is required in the recovery room than in the intensive care unit.

The period between closure of the skin incision and stabilization of the patient in the recovery room can be a hazardous one. To reiterate, attention is often relaxed, monitors are generally disconnected and the patient is transferred to a bed and then over a varying distance to the care of new personnel relatively unfamiliar with the immediate individual problems. Before leaving the operating room, the recovery room should be notified so that necessary equipment and medication can be prepared before the patient arrives.

Careful transfer of the patient must be emphasized. Allowing the patient to resume spontaneous respiration at this time, with the possibility of associated hypercarbia, hypoxemia and anxiety, and restlessness, can be especially dangerous to the patient with heart disease. He may best be transferred with endotracheal tube *in situ* and under anesthesia. If the patient is stable, the pulse can reasonably be the main means of monitoring the circulatory status during transfer. If there have been problems with the blood pressure or rhythm, then pressure and the ECG should also be monitored. Appropriate drugs should be carried with the patient.

Immediately upon arriving in the recovery room, all monitors utilized during the operative period should be reconnected; in a patient with heart disease, these would include an ECG, a blood pressure cuff (or arterial pressure line), and an intravenous line (or a central venous line). Urinary collection bags should be emptied and hourly monitoring begun. Supplemental humidified oxygen should be delivered to the patient with a face mask or endotracheal tube if the patient is spontaneously breathing or by a ventilator if respiration is assisted or controlled. Baseline values should be recorded for cardiac, respiratory, and renal function.

It is imperative that a standard procedure exist for transferring information regarding the nature of the operation, the fluids, blood, and drugs given, the general circulatory state, the anticipated complications, and the plan for immediate management. The anesthetist must remain until the patient's general condition has been established and stabilized.

The patient whose circulatory status is in question is initially left lying flat in bed. When his general condition is established and found satisfactory, the head of the bed may be raised to 30 degrees. The patient should be rolled from side to side every 2 hours to assist in the prevention of basal atelectasis and pulmonary complications.

ACCURATE ASSESSMENT OF THE CARDIOVASCULAR STATUS

Two levels of intensity of assessment of the circulatory status can be defined in patients with heart disease. A relatively simple regimen is adequate following minor procedures in patients who maintain compensated myocardial and pulmonary function. A more intensive assessment regimen is required after major surgical procedures in patients with poor preoperative myocardial or pulmonary function or those whose circulatory status has been unstable intraoperatively.

Routine Assessment Regimen

Myocardial function can be adequately assessed in the majority of patients on purely clinical evidence (Fig. 1). The critical point is to take the time to establish baseline criteria to which change may be compared and upon which subsequent judgment can be based.

The blood pressure can be measured with a sphygmomanometer. The use of a Doppler greatly facilitates identifying the systolic blood pressure in obese or vasoconstricted patients. An electrocardiographic oscilloscope should be connected via stick-on electrodes and the rhythm noted. If any question of electrocardiographic abnormalities is detected, a full ECG should be obtained. The pulse rate should be recorded: a single

ROUTINE ASSESSMENT REGIME

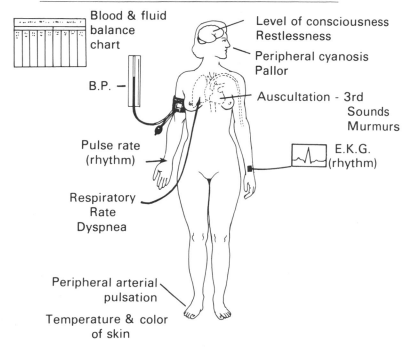

Blood & fluid balance chart

B.P. —

Pulse rate (rhythm)

Respiratory Rate Dyspnea

Peripheral arterial pulsation

Temperature & color of skin

Level of consciousness
Restlessness

Peripheral cyanosis
Pallor

Auscultation - 3rd
Sounds
Murmurs

E.K.G.
(rhythm)

Figure 1. Routine assessment of myocardial function utilized in the postoperative care of the patient with heart disease who has undergone relatively minor procedures and who maintains compensated myocardial and pulmonary function.

rate if the patient is in sinus rhythm, but both apical and radial rates separately in patients in atrial fibrillation. The pulse deficit, the difference between apical and radial rates, records the number of ineffective ventricular contractions.

The heart and lungs should be auscultated in every patient with a history of heart disease. The presence or absence of murmurs should be noted. The presence of a third heart sound (diastolic gallop) suggests ventricular failure. Pulmonary congestion and edema is manifest by crepitation at the bases. Unsuspected pulmonary complications (pneumothorax, basal atelectasis, endotracheal tube malposition) may be detected early if routine auscultation is a part of the clinical examination in the recovery room. In the spontaneously breathing patient,

POSTOPERATIVE CARE   177 rapid shallow breathing should suggest stiff lungs, which are often associated with cardiac failure and a raised left atrial pressure or with pulmonary arterial pressure elevation.

The temperature and color of the skin of the face, knees, and feet, and the level on the legs to which warmth extends should be noted. A low cardiac output is almost always associated with cool vasoconstricted extremities. All major pulses should be palpated: carotid, brachial, radial, femoral, posterior tibial, and dorsalis pedis. In the presence of a low cardiac output with peripheral vasoconstriction, distal pulses are frequently absent; decreased body temperature is not the only cause of their absence postoperatively.

The level of consciousness, state of the pupils, and movement of all limbs should be noted. All restlessness in the patient with heart disease must be assumed to be caused by hypoxemia until proved otherwise.

A blood and fluid balance chart (including the intraoperative values) must be begun at the time of admission to the recovery room and continued diligently until the patient is discharged. It is impossible to establish retrospectively how much volume a patient has received through the perioperative period after a crisis has arisen.

If deterioration is suspected, one should insert a central venous catheter, pass a urinary catheter, and obtain central venous and arterial blood samples for analysis. In this manner, a full intensive assessment regimen is begun by steps, as indicated. Careful observation is the order of the day so that appropriate physiologic values relating to myocardial and peripheral vascular function can be obtained and therapy instituted.

Intensive Assessment Regimen

In addition to the methods employed in routine evaluation, the patient with cardiac decompensation or the patient who deteriorates in the postoperative period must be intensively assessed (Fig. 2).

MYOCARDIUM

Left and right atrial and arterial pressures and cardiac output should be measured. Myocardial contractility can be indirectly assessed by calculating stroke work index and relating this value to the filling pressures. Combined with auscultation, the

INTENSIVE ASSESSMENT REGIME

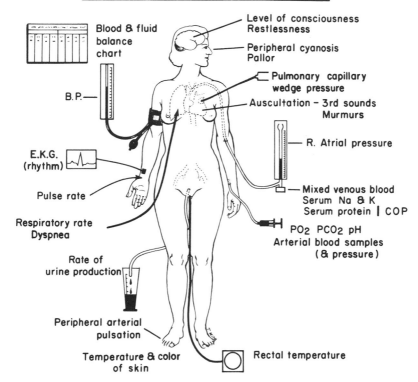

Blood & fluid balance chart

Level of consciousness
Restlessness

Peripheral cyanosis
Pallor

Pulmonary capillary wedge pressure

Auscultation – 3rd sounds
Murmurs

B.P.—

R. Atrial pressure

E.K.G. (rhythm)

Pulse rate

Mixed venous blood
Serum Na & K
Serum protein | COP

Respiratory rate
Dyspnea

PO₂ PCO₂ pH
Arterial blood samples
(& pressure)

Rate of urine production

Peripheral arterial pulsation

Temperature & color of skin

Rectal temperature

Figure 2. Intensive assessment utilized in the postoperative care of the patient with heart disease who has undergone major surgical procedures and evidenced poor myocardial or pulmonary function or whose circulatory status remains questionable. The intensive assessment regimen includes, in addition to the parameters routinely assessed, monitoring the systemic arterial pressure, the central venous and pulmonary arterial occlusion pressures, the arterial and mixed venous oxygen tensions, the arterial carbon dioxide tension and pH, the serum protein concentration or colloid osmotic pressure, the urinary output, and the rectal temperature.

ECG, and evidence of adequate perfusion of the skin and other organs, these physiologic variables allow a reasonably precise indication of the state of the myocardium.

Ideally, both right and left (pulmonary artery occlusion) atrial pressures should be measured. The filling pressure of each ventricle is critical to its optimum function, and disparate function is common in critically ill surgical patients.[1]

These central pressures can be measured through lines inserted by a variety of routes and utilizing a variety of techniques. The most important aspect of invasive monitoring in general is to develop the facility for routine placement; central lines cannot be reserved for only the already acutely ill, as the information gained has its greatest chance of changing the course of disease if used in a prophylactic manner. The pressures must be measured with transducers as the dynamic trace allows the wave form and the pulse pressure to be visualized. Saline manometers are effective in the unconscious paralyzed patient, but give only an approximation of mean pressures. An accurate zero and frequent calibration are required if the pressures are to give useful information.

The cardiac output can be directly measured either by dye or thermal dilution. A clinically useful assessment of flow can also be estimated using either central venous or pulmonary arterial blood gases. Clinically, a simplified Fick equation can be used for this purpose.[2] The total quantity of *oxygen available* for tissue consumption in a given time must include the arterial oxygen content (CaO_2) multiplied by the quantity of blood (the cardiac output—$\dot{Q}_t$) presented to the tissues in a given period of time. The quantity of *oxygen returned* to the lungs is expressed as the total cardiac output multiplied by the mixed venous oxygen content ($C_v\text{-}O_2$). Therefore, the tissue oxygen consumption ($\dot{V}O_2$) must equal the oxygen that has been extracted from the blood, i.e., the difference between the oxygen available and the oxygen returned:

$$\dot{V}O_2 = (\dot{Q}_T)\,(CaO_2) - (\dot{Q}_T)\,(C_v\text{-}O_2).$$

This equation can be simplified and rewritten as

$$\dot{Q}_T = \frac{\dot{V}O_2}{(CaO_2 - C_v\text{-}O_2)}$$

It must be emphasized that mixed venous oxygen content can be accurately measured only in the pulmonary artery. However, venous blood obtained from the superior and inferior vena cavae can also be used to reflect oxygen extraction. The myocardial blood supply is the most marginal of any organ, even under normal conditions, when compared with its metabolic oxygen demand (A-Vo$_2$ difference). The coronary sinus empties directly into the right atrium, and blood samples taken from catheters with the tip in the right atrium show tremendous variation from sample to sample because of the channeling of blood from various sources. Shapiro and coworkers[3] have shown that in human subjects at rest, venous samples taken simultaneously from a catheter in the superior vena cava and the pulmonary artery give reasonably close values. They have also demonstrated that although the relationship became less well defined in the critically ill patient, it was sufficiently predictable to act as a reliable trend indicator. Clinically, if either the pulmonary artery or superior vena cava PaO$_2$ falls below 30 to 35 torr, cardiovascular decompensation must be presumed and the appropriate therapeutic steps initiated.

Arterial cannulation for management of arterial blood pressure and blood gas is now commonplace. The insertion of a cannula in the artery carries the possibility of thrombosis or arterial spasm, which are of little significance if the palmar arch is supplied by an ulnar artery. The presence of the ulnar artery can be established by direct palpation or exsanguination of the hand by having the patient make a fist and noting if the hand flushes on release with the radial artery occluded (Allen test).[4] Most peripheral arteries have from time to time had their advocates for use as a site for placement of arterial cannulae. Other factors appear more important than site in preventing complications. These include judicious attention so that air and foreign material are not injected (peripheral embolization), frequent or continuous infusion of a heparinized isotonic solution, use of small catheters in relation to the size of the artery, and removal of the catheter at the first sign of distal circulatory compromise.

LUNGS

Deterioration of respiratory function in the patient with heart disease, especially in the patient with pre-existing chronic lung disease, is common. There is an increase in the alveolar-arterial oxygen gradient P(A-a)O$_2$ during general anesthesia that persists into the postoperative period regardless of the type of surgery or its magnitude.[5] Levels of oxygenation postoperatively are unpredictable. Hypoxemia may be caused by either a reduction in alveolar oxygen tension or by a defect in the gas-exchanging capacity of the lung itself. The major clinical causes of hypoxemia are (1) hypoventilation (normal $P(A-a)O_2$), (2) ventilation-perfusion mismatch (increased $P(A-a)O_2$ with F_IO_2 = .21), and (3) shunt (increased $P(A-a)O_2$ on all F_IO_2). Pure hypoventilation is associated with a normal $P(A-a)O_2$, while shunt and ventilation-perfusion mismatch are associated with an abnormal $P(A-a)O_2$. Hypoxemia caused by hypoventilation and ventilation-perfusion mismatch can be reversed with relatively low concentrations of oxygen (30 to 35 percent), while hypoxemia caused by shunt may be refractory to oxygen therapy. The major point to remember is that if PaO_2 improves markedly on low concentrations of oxygen, the most likely diagnosis is ventilation-perfusion mismatching. If the PaO_2 is relatively resistant to low concentrations of oxygen, then shunt is the most likely cause of the hypoxemia and further diagnostic and therapeutic efforts are indicated. It should be emphasized that a low mixed venous-oxygen tension will increase the $P(A-a)O_2$.

The postoperative additive effects of central depression from anesthetic agents, the neuromuscular defects from muscle relaxants, and the splinting effect of abdominal or thoracic pain further interfere with an already compromised ventilatory system. Frequent monitoring of arterial blood gases is imperative in addition to the already stressed evaluation of physical signs by auscultation and by noting respiratory rate and pattern. A chest x-ray is also usually taken within a few hours of the patient's return from the operating room if cardiac disease is suspected.

KIDNEYS

Urinary production is monitored by inserting a catheter into the bladder and recording the volume produced per hour. While renal function is not the topic of this chapter, urinary volume serves as one indicator of renal blood flow and thus as a guide to cardiac output and peripheral perfusion. While normal urinary flow does not necessarily indicate good renal function, oliguria can only occur if renal function is depressed.

BODY CHEMISTRY

The biochemical problems that most frequently concern the anesthetist in the postoperative period are essentially simple. Of concern are the red cells, which carry oxygen; plasma, which upholds the colloid osmotic pressure and sustains the blood pressure; sodium, which is the osmotic particle that maintains the fluid content of the extracellular space; potassium, which is primarily noted for its special effects on cardiac electrical conduction; and acid-base balance, which is so dependent on buffering mechanisms and so easily upset by acute physiologic deterioration and by the anesthetist's intervention.[6]

BODY TEMPERATURE

Normal heat-regulating mechanisms are compromised postoperatively. Cardiac irregularities occur at or about 30°C body temperature, although they may be present earlier if there is any retention of CO_2 or electrolytic abnormality. The metabolism of certain anesthetic drugs may not continue at a normothermic rate, and therefore they exert their effects long into the postoperative period. Nondepolarizing muscle relaxants produce demonstrable effects up to 12 hours after their administration.[7] Neostigmine, the drug commonly used for reversal of these relaxants, has a relatively short duration of action. This fact becomes especially pertinent in the cold patient, who may not have metabolized the muscle relaxants to the usual degree by the end of the operative procedure. The resultant "recurarization," with decreased respiratory exchange coupled with the increased oxygen requirements caused by shivering in the postoperative period, gives rise to a highly dangerous situation. Dramatic decreases in body temperature must be corrected.

PREVENTION AND TREATMENT OF COMPLICATIONS

The touchstone of therapy in the patient with heart disease is early detection. The differential diagnosis of low cardiac output includes all the parameters discussed in the routine and intensive assessment regimens. The anesthetist's goals while managing the patient postoperatively reduce to preserving and increasing what reserve potential exists, providing early warning of impending failure by diligent and frequent observation, and instituting progressively more intensive monitoring if instability is suspected.

Even in the patient whose heart disease is confined to the coronary arteries, the chance that the stress of anesthesia and surgery may precipitate cardiac decompensation increases.[8] The same is true for patients with other types of heart disease. Those with established rheumatic or hypertensive cardiac disease may first experience congestive heart failure during the intra- and postoperative periods. Brockner[9] studied 235 patients between 60 and 89 years of age, 166 of whom were operated on for carcinoma of the stomach. Among those with cardiac symptoms, electrocardiographic changes suggesting degeneration, an enlarged heart revealed by x-ray, and no preoperative digitalis, one half required postoperative digitalization. Deutsch[10] recommends administering digitalis before any major operation when there is a history of cardiac symptoms or electrocardiographic changes suggestive of degeneration or when enlargement of the heart has been demonstrated radiologically. The importance of marginal cardiac function cannot be overemphasized.[11] Digitalization should be maintained throughout the perioperative period. Although the exact place of prophylactic digitalization has not yet been established, there is an ever-increasing tendency to provide this background of positive inotropic support in the compensated heart disease patient. The awareness that levels of serum potassium must be maintained and that doses of digitalis considerably smaller than the usual "digitalizing" dose produce significant hemodynamic effect has led to an increase in the margin of safety in the use of digitalis, particularly in the patient without overt failure.[12] The increased margin of cardiac reserve afforded by prophylactic digitalization has recently received added support through studies in animals that demonstrate protection against the depression in contractile force caused by both pentobarbital anesthesia and hemorrhagic shock. [13, 14]

Myocardial Infarction

A patient with a history of myocardial infarction, specifically if it occurred in the previous 6 months, has an increased chance of cardiac death after general anesthesia for noncardiac operations.[15] Analysis of factors leading to myocardial infarction and heart failure in the postoperative period seems to support the thesis developed by Braunwald and Moroko,[16] who produced either reduction or augmentation of infarct size by influencing the balance between myocardial oxygen supply and demand. Postoperative myocardial infarction and heart failure or cardiogenic shock, both complications with impressively high mortality rates, occur more frequently in patients (1) with advanced coronary artery disease, indicated by arterial hypertension or cerebral vascular and arterial occlusive disease or present or past heart failure, (2) after reduction of myocardial oxygen supply, indicated by hypotension during anesthesia or anemia in the perioperative period, and (3) in coincidence with an elevated oxygen demand predominantly during the early postoperative period when catecholamines are increased.

It is also important to note that primary postoperative infarction or reinfarction is a highly lethal disease; 54 percent mortality was reported in a series from the Mayo Clinic.[17] It must be stressed that patients who have had a previous infarction fall into the group who must be intensely assessed throughout the perioperative period. Supplemental oxygen provides significant hemodynamic effects following myocardial infarction.[18] Daily electrocardiograms for comparison with preoperative ones are needed to detect "silent" infarctions.

The specific choice of therapy for the patient who develops myocardial decompensation lies beyond the scope of this chapter. The point that again bears re-emphasizing is that prophylaxis is the order of the day and judicious monitoring the primary concern.

Respiratory Complications

Respiratory complications in the patient with heart disease, especially in patients with pre-existing chronic lung disease, remain a difficult problem. It is especially important to emphasize the place of postoperative chest physiotherapy in this group of patients. Various mechanical devices such as intermittent positive-pressure breathing, rebreathing tubes, water bottles, incentive spirometers, and endotracheal catheters have been proposed to assist in the postoperative respiratory care of the patient with borderline cardiac function. The patient who can cough effectively but whose efforts are diminished because of pain or residual anesthesia can indeed be benefited by a wide variety of approaches. The patient who cannot raise his secretions, however, must be attended by active nursing involvement, including endotracheal suctioning and chest physiotherapy; as yet there are no mechanical devices capable of replacing these specific therapeutic modalities.[19]

Fortunately, in the seriously ill patient with underlying heart disease, mechanical support of ventilation has few limitations and many advantages. Elective, short-term, intermittent positive-pressure ventilation should, therefore, be considered after all major operations in the patient with heart disease, and longer-term support, i.e., 24 to 48 hours or longer, is mandatory in the critically ill. Ventilatory support in the immediate postoperative period provides effective control of alveolar ventilation at a time when cardiac output may be either depressed or labile. Any reduction in cardiac output at this time magnifies the effects of the venous admixture from intrapulmonary shunts created by closure of small airways or ventilation-perfusion inequalities. To reiterate, the increased A-aDO$_2$ manifest following general anesthesia has multiple etiologies. Increased pulmonary venous admixture, caused by either true shunt or changes in distribution of ventilation-perfusion ratios within the lung, together with changes in cardiac output are contributory factors. The degree of reduction in cardiac output necessary to produce such changes is not uncommon during and following anesthesia.

Since 1955 when Bjork and Engstrom[20] first described the successful use of mechanical ventilation following pulmonary resection, the principle of postoperative artificial ventilation in cases at high risk of developing pulmonary insufficiency has been increasingly accepted. Bauman[21] succeeded in preventing postoperative pulmonary complications by elective ventilation of patients following thoracic surgery. He proposed a period of postoperative elective ventilation in patients with preoperative respiratory or cardiac factors likely to give rise to respiratory insufficiency. Thus, adequate analgesia can be provided without fear of interference with adequacy of ventilation. Postoperative pulmonary complications are likely to be prevented in this group of patients when adequate lung function is maintained and oxygenation can be controlled.[22]

CONCLUSION

The seriously ill patient with heart disease in the hands of a highly trained and conscientious anesthetist is certainly more likely to have a benign course during and after surgery today than in the past. Although it lies outside the scope of this chapter to detail the specific management of all aspects of cardiac disease, it must be re-emphasized that the touchstone of therapy lies in routine and progressive intensive assessment.

REFERENCES

1. Civetta, J. M., Gabel, J. C., and Laver, M. B.: *Disparate ventricular function in surgical patients.* Surg. Forum 22, 1971.
2. Scher, A. M.: "Control of arterial blood pressure: measurement of pressure and flow." In Ruch, T. C., and Pattan, H. D.: *Physiology and Biophysics.* W. B. Saunders, Philadelphia, 1965, p. 680.
3. Shapiro, B. A.: *Blood gas interpretations in critically ill patients.* Respir. Care 21:507, 1976.
4. Allen, E. V.: *Thromboangiitis obliterans: methods of diagnosis of chronic occlusive arterial lesions distal to the wrist with illustrative cases.* Am. J. Med. Sci. 178:237, 1929.
5. Panday, J., and Nunn, J. F.: *Failure to demonstrate progressive falls of arterial PO$_2$ during anesthesia.* Anesthesia 23:38, 1968.
6. Gabel, J. C.: "Biochemical monitoring." In Saidman, L. J., and Smith, N. T. (eds.): *Monitoring in Anesthesia.* John Wiley & Sons, New York, pp. 15–29.
7. Hannington-Kiff, J. G.: *Residual post-operative paralysis.* Proc. R. Soc. Med. 63:73, 1970.
8. Mushin, W. W.: *The normality of the abnormal.* Anesth. Analg. (Cleve.) 49:667, 1970.
9. Brockner, J.: *The evaluation of surgical patients for pre-operative digitalization.* Acta Chir. Scand. 129:1, 1965.
10. Deutsch, S., and Dalen, J. E.: *Indications for prophylactic digitalization.* Anesthesiology 30:648, 1969.
11. Goldman, L.: *Multifactorial index of cardiac risk in non-cardiac surgical procedures.* N. Engl. J. Med. 297:845, 1977.
12. Weissler, A. M., Snyder, J. R., Schoenfeld, C. D., et al.: *Assay of digitalis glycosides in man.* Am. J. Cardiol. 17:768, 1966.
13. Crowell, J. S., and Smith, E. E.: *Oxygen dificit and irreversible hemorrhagic shock.* Am. J. Physiol. 206:313, 1968.
14. Merchants, F. J., Feinberg, H., and Levitsky, S.: *Reversal of myocardial depression by dipyridamole following aortic cross-clamping.* Surg. Forum 23:162, 1972.
15. Goldman, L., Caldera, D. L., Southwick, F. S., et al.: *Cardiac risk factors and complications in non-cardiac surgery.* Medicine 57:357, 1978.
16. Braunwald, E., and Moroko, P. R.: *The reduction of infarct size—an idea whose time (for testing) has come.* Circulation 50:206, 1974.

17. Tarhan, S., Moffitt, E. A., Taylor, W. F., et al.: *Myocardial infarction after general anesthesia.* J.A.M.A. 220, 1451, 1972.
18. Daly, W. J., and Bondurant, S.: *Effects of oxygen breathing on the heart rate, blood pressure, and cardiac index of normal men —resting, with reactive hyperemia, and after atropine.* J. Clin. Invest. 41:126, 1962.
19. Tarhan, S., Moffitt, E. A., Sessler, A. D., et al.: *Risk of anesthesia and surgery in patients with chronic bronchitis and chronic obstructive pulmonary disease.* Surgery 74:720, 1973.
20. Bjork, V. O., and Engstrom, C. G.: *The treatment of ventilatory insufficiency after pulmonary resection with tracheostomy and prolonged artificial ventilation.* J. Thorac. Surg. 30:356, 1955.
21. Baumann, J., Pogart, C. L., and Stieglitz, P.: *Prevention and treatment of post-operative respiratory insufficiency in lung surgery by means of respiratory assistance without tracheostomy.* Ann. Chir. Thorac. Cardiovasc. 3:125, 1961.
22. Gerson, G.: *Pre-operative respiratory function tests and post-operative mortality (a study of patients undergoing surgery for carcinoma of the bronchus).* Br. J. Anaesth. 41:967, 1969.

INDEX

Morphine
  aortic stenosis and, 46
  tetrad spell and, 50
Mustard procedure, 54
Myocardial infarction
  intraoperative recurrence of,
    hypotension and, 61
  measurement of, 79–80
  postoperative, 57–63, 184–185
    recurrence of, duration of
      anesthesia and, 61–62
    hypertension and, 61
    preoperative factors and, 62
    site of operation and, 61
    timing of, 60
  reduction of, 80–81
  surgical postponement and,
    62–63
Myocardial ischemia
  anesthetic risk in, 69–72
  electrocardiogram and, 21–22
  intraoperative management of,
    75–79
  preoperative evaluation of, 72–75
    contractility in, 73
    drug therapy in, 73–75
    myocardial perfusion in, 72–73

NARCOTICS, coronary artery disease
    and, 77
Neuroleptanesthesia, ventricular
    function and, 11
Neuromuscular blocking drugs,
    ventricular function and,
    11–12
Nitroglycerin
  coronary artery disease and, 66
  ischemic myocardium and, 81
  preoperative, 75
Nitroprusside
  ischemic myocardium and, 81
  recovery room hypertension and,
    99
Nitrous oxide
  coronary artery disease and,
    78–79
  hypotension and, 109
  ventricular function and, 9, 14
Nitrous oxide-oxygen-muscle
    relaxant sequence, aortic
    stenosis and, 46
Node, atrioventricular, conduction
    delay in, 127–129
Nuclear cardiology, 24

OXYGEN, myocardial consumption
    of, 103–107
Oxygenation
  arterial, 34
  postoperative measurement of,
    180–182
  tetrad spell and, 50

P WAVE, 21
Pancuronium, 77
Patent ductus arteriosus, 43
Pediatric heart patient,
    psychological status of, 56
Perfusion, myocardial, 12–13,
    72–73
Pneumocardiography, 24
Potassium (K+), low serum,
    preoperative digitalis and, 75
Preload, ventricular function and,
    3–5
Premature beats, isolated, 149–154
Pressure
  central venous, 4–5, 24–25
  elevated airway, hypotension and,
    112–113
  pulmonary artery occluded, left
    ventricular function and, 4–5
Prognosis, postoperative, in
    patients with pre-existing
    heart disease, 57–63
Propranidid, ventricular function
    and, 10
Propranolol
  hypertension and, 96
  infarct size and, 80
  preoperative use of, 73–74
  tetrad spell and, 50
Pulmonary valve
  absence of, 46–48
  insufficiency of, 46–48
  stenosis of, 46

RASHKIND procedure, 54
Rate-pressure product, 105
Recovery room as intensive care
    area, 174–175
Relaxants, intraoperative
    hypotension and, 77
Respiration, postoperative
    assessment of, 181–182
    complications of, 185–186
Respiratory distress syndrome, 43
Rhythm. See also Arrhythmia,
    Bradyarrhythmia, Premature